BASIC SKILLS

Health, Hygiene and Safety

Di Barton and Wilf Stout

D0513094

JOHN MURRAY

Other books in the Basic Skills series:
English by Paul Groves and Nigel Grimshaw
with *Teachers' Resource Book*
Arithmetic by John Deft
with *Teachers' Resource Book*
Science by Peter Leckstein
Electronics by Tom Duncan
Geography by Sally Naish and Katherine Goldsmith
with *Teachers' Resource Book*

A related book on life skills:
Lifestart by John Anderson

First published 1988
by John Murray (Publishers) Ltd
50 Albemarle Street, London W1X 4BD

Reprinted 1992 (with revisions), 1995, 1997

Printed and bound in Great Britain
at The Bath Press, Bath

British Library Cataloguing in Publication Data

Barton, Di.
  Basic skills.
  1. Man. Health   2. Man. Hygiene – For Schools
  3. Safety
  I. Title   II. Stout, G.W. (G. Wilf)
  613

  ISBN 0–7195–4463–7

About this Book

In this book we deal with three areas of science that everyone needs to know about and understand:

Personal Health is about how the body works, ways of keeping healthy, and problems of emotional well-being, addiction and handicaps.

Hygiene and Community Health is concerned with food preservation and hygiene, infectious diseases and hazards like pollution and noise.

Safety deals with protection from dangers at home, on the roads and at work.

The content is designed for those studying for the AEB's *Basic Test* in *Health, Hygiene and Safety*. We hope however that it will prove useful to the many other students at school and college who need a grounding in these important areas.

Contents

PERSONAL HEALTH
Unit 1 How the Body Works

You should understand the basic facts about how your body works and how each system functions, so that you can maintain your own good health and look after your body. You should also know something about your emotional, as well as physical, well-being and understand how to cope with stress in your life.

What are you really made of?

Your body is made of about 50 billion tiny **cells**. There are different types of cell, with different structures to allow them to do different jobs in the body. For example, nerve cells carry messages, skin cells protect the body and red blood cells carry oxygen.

Most of the cells in the body are grouped together to form **tissues**. This helps the cells to carry out their particular function more efficiently. For example, the large muscle in your upper arm, the biceps, is made up of millions of tiny muscle cells which contract and enable you to lift your forearm.

Several different tissues combine together to form **organs** such as the heart and stomach. Groups of organs work together as **organ systems**, for example the heart, blood vessels and blood form the circulatory system, the mouth, stomach, intestines and rectum form the digestive system.

cells ⟶ tissues ⟶ organs ⟶ organ systems

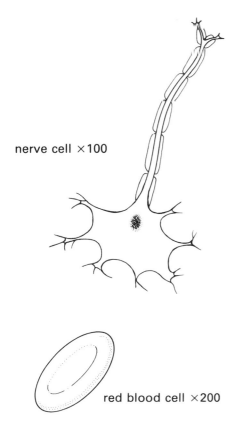

nerve cell ×100

red blood cell ×200

These are just two of the different types of cells found in the body. Notice how different they are in shape and size.

All the cells, tissues, organs and organ systems in our bodies have special jobs, and work together to keep us fit and well.

Notice how cells are grouped together.

(a) Single muscle cells

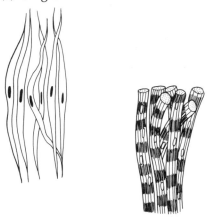

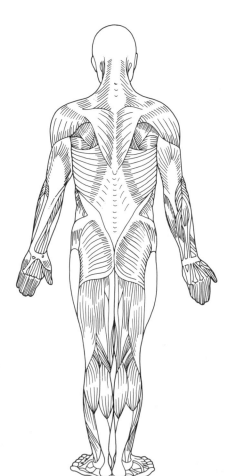

(b) Groups of muscle cells forming tissues

(c) Positions of muscle tissues in the body

How is your body organized?

You have seven main organ systems in your body:

1. the **digestive system** supplies food to your body,
2. the **respiratory system** supplies oxygen and removes carbon dioxide,
3. the **circulatory system** carries food and oxygen to every cell,
4. the **skeletal system** supports your body and works with the muscles to move your body,
5. the **excretory system** removes harmful waste produced by your body,
6. the **reproductive system** enables you to produce a baby,
7. the **nervous system** collects information and controls all the organ systems.

---

1 What type of cell carries oxygen round the body?
2 What are groups of similar cells called?
3 Name one example of an organ.
4 Which organ system provides food to the body?
5 What is the function of the respiratory system?

The digestive system

How does food get into your body?

We all need food to stay alive. Your whole body is made up of materials which you have eaten at some time in your life. The food that you eat is made up mainly of carbohydrates, proteins and fats which are taken into your digestive system as molecules. Molecules are the smallest forms in which each of these chemical substances can exist. However, even these molecules are too big to get out of your digestive system and into your circulatory system, so they have to be broken down. The breakdown of large molecules of food into smaller molecules in the digestive system is called **digestion**.

Digestion begins in your mouth with your teeth cutting and chewing food into small pieces. During this time the food gets covered in a liquid called saliva produced by salivary glands in the mouth. Saliva makes the food

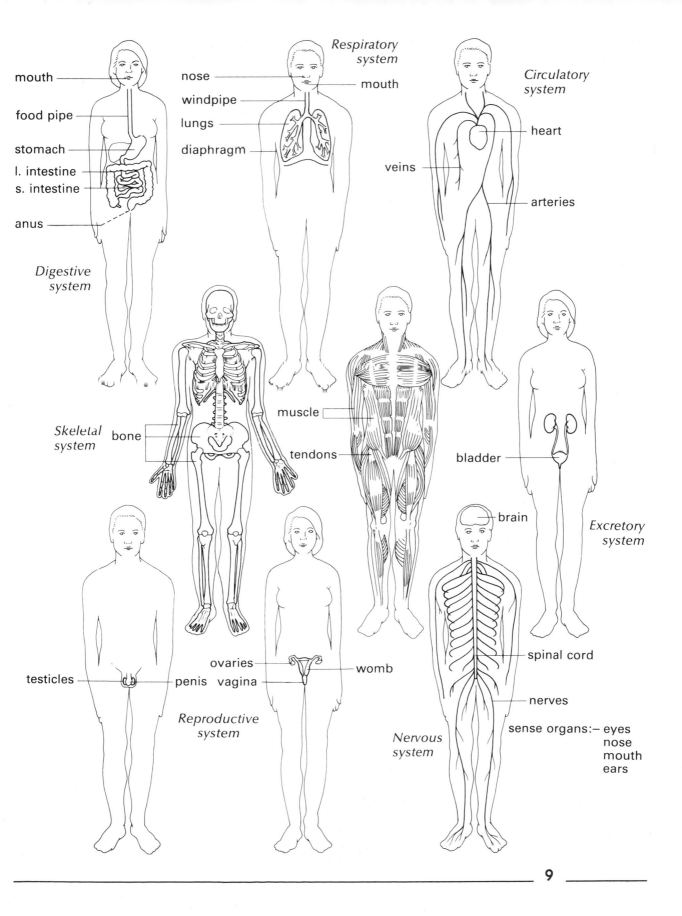

mouth

food pipe

stomach

l. intestine

s. intestine

anus

*Digestive
system*

nose

windpipe

lungs

diaphragm

*Respiratory
system*

mouth

*Circulatory
system*

heart

veins

arteries

*Skeletal
system*　bone

muscle

tendons

bladder

*Excretory
system*

testicles

penis

ovaries

vagina

womb

*Reproductive
system*

brain

spinal cord

nerves

sense organs:- eyes
nose
mouth
ears

*Nervous
system*

wet and easy to swallow. It also contains a chemical which helps to break down large molecules of starch in your food into small molecules of a sugar called glucose. Chemicals which help the body to break down large molecules to small molecules are called **enzymes.**

When you swallow your food it passes down through your oesophagus to your stomach where it stays for about three hours. The cells in your stomach produce an acidic liquid called gastric juice. An enzyme in gastric juice starts the breakdown of large molecules of protein into small molecules called amino acids. This enzyme will only work in the presence of an acid which is the reason why your stomach produces acid. If your stomach produces too much acid you will suffer from indigestion.

Enzymes break down starch to glucose.

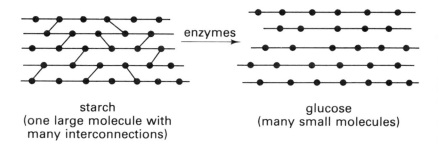

starch
(one large molecule with many interconnections)

glucose
(many small molecules)

After your food has been partly digested it is ready to move to the next part of the digestive system. To do this a muscular valve at the end of the stomach relaxes and the food is squirted into the **small intestine.**

Your small intestine is where most of the digestion of food takes place. It is about 6 metres long. The first 30 centimetres is called the duodenum and the latter part is called the ileum. The cells of the duodenum and a gland called the pancreas found close to it produce digestive enzymes to break down starch, proteins and fats. The liver also releases a chemical liquid called bile which helps the enzymes to break down fats.

The muscles in the wall of the small intestine contract and relax and squeeze the food along the duodenum. Digestion occurs in the duodenum and the ileum and all the large molecules of food are broken down into small molecules. These pass through the cells of the wall of the digestive system into the blood stream by a process called **absorption.**

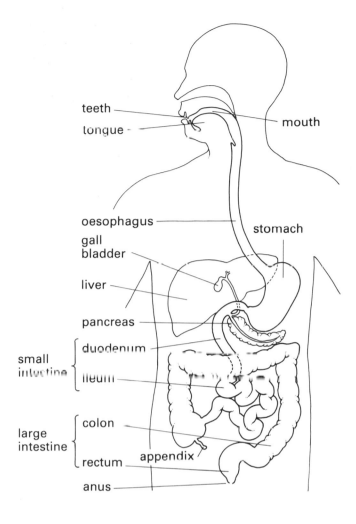

The digestive system.

teeth

tongue

mouth

oesophagus

stomach

gall bladder

liver

pancreas

duodenum

small intestine

ileum

large intestine

colon

rectum

appendix

anus

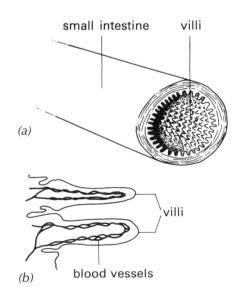

small intestine   villi

(a)

villi

blood vessels

(b)

The small intestine is where food is absorbed into the blood.
(a) Villi in the small intestine.
(b) Blood vessels in the villi.

The small intestine has a very large surface area so that it can absorb as many food molecules as possible. The surface area of the intestine is about 300 square metres, that is, larger than a tennis court. In the wall of the small intestine there are thousands of tiny finger-like structures called villi which have a very good supply of small blood vessels (capillaries). These take away the food molecules from the digestive system and pass them quickly to the rest of the body.

The undigested food and other waste products which are left in the small intestine then pass into the **large intestine**. This is made up of the colon, where water is absorbed, and the rectum. The remaining waste, called faeces, is then passed out of the body through the rectum and anus.

If the faeces move too quickly through your large intestine not enough water is absorbed and the faeces become too runny and soft and cause you to have diarrhoea. If the faeces are moved too slowly through your large intestine too much water is absorbed and the faeces become dry and hard. This will cause you to be constipated.

An adequate amount of fibre in your everyday diet helps you to pass faeces out at regular intervals.

---

1 Why do large molecules of food have to be digested?
2 Name the chemicals which break down large molecules to small molecules.
3 What type of food is broken down in the stomach?
4 Where does the digestion of protein first begin?
5 What causes indigestion?
6 How is food moved along the digestive system?
7 How is the surface area of the small intestine increased?
8 What happens in the large intestine?
9 How does constipation occur?
10 How can you prevent constipation?

The respiratory system

How does oxygen get into your body?

All the cells in your body need **oxygen** to release **energy** from food and they obtain this oxygen from the air. About one fifth of the air around you is oxygen, the rest is nitrogen.

You can't beat fresh country air!

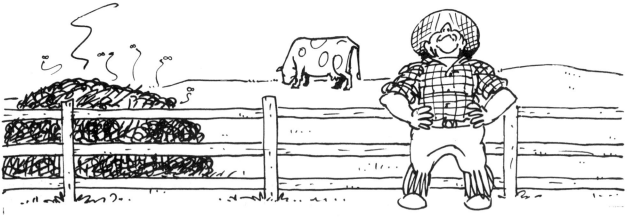

How do you breathe in?

Try taking a deep breath. Can you feel your chest becoming larger? This is caused by the muscles between your ribs contracting to move your ribs upwards and outwards. At the same time a flat muscle across the base of your ribs also contracts and moves downwards. This flat muscle is called the **diaphragm**. The movements of the ribs and the diaphragm *increase* the volume of your chest and *reduce* the pressure of the air inside your lungs. Air in the atmosphere which is at a higher pressure than that in your lungs rushes into the lungs to balance the difference in pressure.

Where does the oxygen go?

When air moves in through your nose some of the dust particles are filtered out by the hairs in your nose. The air is also warmed and moistened. From your nose the air takes the following route to the lungs:

windpipe ⟶ bronchus ⟶ bronchiole ⟶ air sacs
(trachea)   (alveoli)

This is what happens to the ribs and the diaphragm when you breathe in and out.

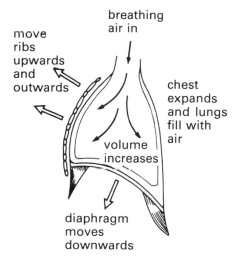

breathing air in

move ribs upwards and outwards

chest expands and lungs fill with air

volume increases

diaphragm moves downwards

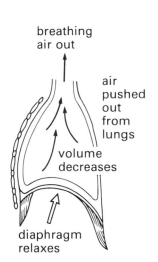

breathing air out

air pushed out from lungs

volume decreases

diaphragm relaxes

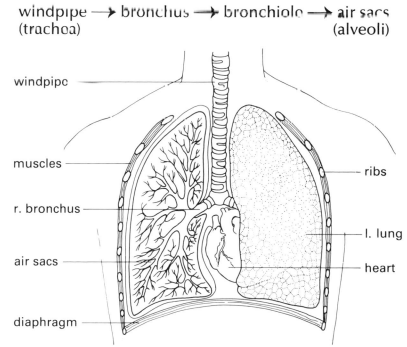

windpipe

muscles

r. bronchus

air sacs

diaphragm

ribs

l. lung

heart

Notice how the lungs, ribs and diaphragm surround the heart.

When it reaches the **air sacs (alveoli)**, the oxygen in the air passes into the blood.

How does the oxygen get into your blood?

You have about 500 million tiny air sacs (alveoli) in your lungs and each of them is covered by many blood

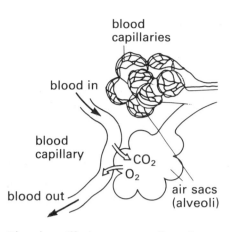

blood capillaries

blood in

blood capillary

CO_2

O_2

blood out

air sacs (alveoli)

Blood capillaries surrounding the air spaces in the air sacs of the lungs. Notice how oxygen (O_2) enters the blood capillary and carbon dioxide (CO_2) leaves.

capillaries. When the air that you have breathed in fills up the air sacs the oxygen molecules inside them move out into the blood in the capillaries, where the oxygen combines with a chemical called **haemoglobin** in the red blood cells.

What happens when you breathe out?

You breathe in and out about twelve times a minute. When you breathe out you can feel your chest cavity getting smaller. The movement of the ribs and diaphragm *reduces* the volume of your chest and *increases* the pressure of the air in your lungs. This forces air out of the body and at the same time an unwanted gas called **carbon dioxide**, moves from the blood capillaries into the air in the air sacs. As you breathe out you remove this unwanted gas from your body.

What makes you cough?

Sometimes crumbs of food can get into your windpipe and these have to be removed by coughing. When you cough the lungs push out a blast of air which shifts the food particle. Any irritation in your windpipe can make you cough, it doesn't have to be food. Sometimes bacteria get into the bronchi and set up an infection, such as a disease called **bronchitis**. When this happens your lungs produce a lot of **phlegm** (mucus) which has to be removed by coughing.

1 How much of the air is oxygen?
2 Why is oxygen needed in your body?
3 Describe two ways you can increase the size of your chest when you breathe in.
4 Why should you breathe through your nose?
5 What are air sacs?
6 How does oxygen get from an air sac into your blood?
7 Which organ pumps blood around your body?
8 What gas is removed when you breathe out?
9 Why do you cough?
10 What is bronchitis?

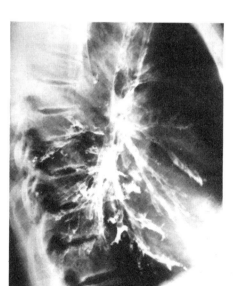

X-ray photograph of a lung of someone suffering from bronchitis.

The circulatory system

What is blood and what does it do?

All through your body are hundreds of fine tubes called blood vessels which carry blood to every cell in your body. The blood carries all the food and oxygen which is needed by your cells.

About half of your blood is a liquid called **plasma** which carries food molecules (such as glucose, amino acids), hormones and waste substances round your body. The other half is made up of red blood cells and white blood cells.

There are about 25 billion red blood cells in your body and their job is to carry oxygen from the blood capillaries of the lungs to every cell in your body. The red blood cells contain haemoglobin which helps them to pick up the oxygen more efficiently. When blood leaves the lungs it contains a high level of oxygen and it is described as being oxygenated.

There are normally about 20 000 million white blood cells in your body. If you are ill these can increase to two or three times that number, as white blood cells help to protect you against disease. One type of white blood cell actually engulfs and destroys bacteria — see the diagram below. Another type of white blood cell produces chemicals called **antibodies** which attack and destroy viruses and bacteria which cause disease.

Red and white blood cells as seen under a microscope.

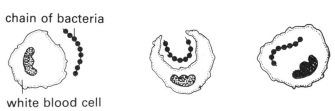

chain of bacteria

white blood cell

A white blood cell engulfing and destroying bacteria.

The blood also contains tiny particles called **platelets** which help your blood to clot if you cut yourself.

How is blood carried around the body?

Blood leaves the heart in blood vessels called **arteries** which have thick muscular walls. Further away from the heart the arteries branch into smaller blood vessels and eventually form a mass of tiny tubes called **capillaries**. Capillaries are found in muscles and in all the organs of the body. It is here that food and oxygen leave the blood and carbon dioxide and waste substances move into the blood from the cells.

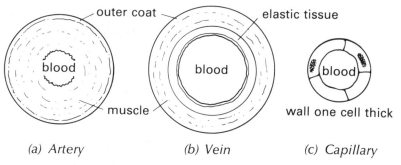

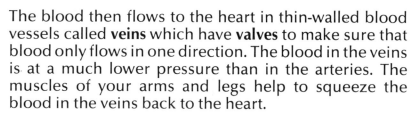

(a) Artery   *(b) Vein*   *(c) Capillary*

Structure of blood vessels (not to scale).

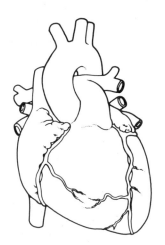

External features of the human heart.

The blood then flows to the heart in thin-walled blood vessels called **veins** which have **valves** to make sure that blood only flows in one direction. The blood in the veins is at a much lower pressure than in the arteries. The muscles of your arms and legs help to squeeze the blood in the veins back to the heart.

How is blood pumped around the body?

The **heart** is a pump which pushes the blood in the blood vessels through the whole of the body.

It is made up of four chambers which fill and empty about 70 times each minute. The two lower chambers are called **ventricles** and they have thick muscular walls which contract to push the blood out of the heart in arteries.

Structure of the heart, showing the positions of the different valves.

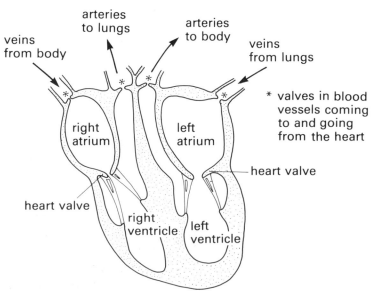

When the ventricles contract:

- Blood from the right side of the heart goes to the lungs where it collects more oxygen before returning to the left side of the heart.
- Blood from the left side of the heart is pumped around the whole body. The muscle of the left ventricle is much thicker than the muscle of the right ventricle as it has to pump the blood further.
- Veins return the blood to the upper chambers which are called **atria** (one is an **atrium**).

When the atria fill up, the blood passes into the ventricles. Valves between the atria and the ventricles stop the blood returning into the atria when the ventricles pump blood into the arteries. There are valves at the base of the arteries to stop the blood returning to the ventricles when the ventricles are filling up with blood from the atria.

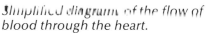

Simplified diagram of the flow of blood through the heart.

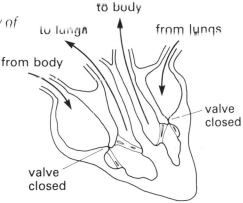
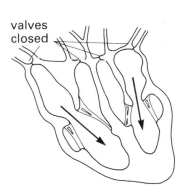

(a) *Both ventricles contract — blood is forced from the ventricles to the lungs and body. At the same time the atria fill up with blood.*

(b) *Both atria contract — blood is forced from the atria to the ventricles.*

Although the heart beats about 70 times a minute, if you are excited or frightened your heart beat increases so that more blood, carrying food and oxygen, reaches the cells. When you are asleep or very relaxed your heart beat slows down as your body does not need so much oxygen.

If the artery carrying blood to the muscle of the heart (the **coronary artery**) gets narrow and stops blood flowing the heart cannot beat and this causes a **heart attack**. Smoking, eating fatty foods and lack of exercise can make a heart attack more likely.

1 Name two substances carried by the plasma.
2 What are the two types of blood cells?
3 What is oxygenated blood?
4 What is the function of the white blood cells?
5 What is the function of the platelets?
6 What type of blood vessels carry blood away from the heart?
7 What happens when the blood reaches the muscles?
8 What two chambers of the heart contract to pump blood away from the heart?
9 Why does the left ventricle have a thicker wall than the right?
10 What is the purpose of the valves in the heart?
11 Name two factors which increase the rate of your heart beat.
12 What should you avoid if you want to prevent a heart attack?

The skeletal system

How does your body move?

You can move your head, waggle your toes, even waggle your ears and twitch your nose. More usefully though, you can move from place to place. This is possible because your muscles and bones work together in such a way to enable you to do these things.

You have about two hundred different bones in your body. The smallest bone is found in your ear and the largest bone is the femur found in the leg. Look at the diagram opposite and see where the main bones in the body are found.

Bones support your body and protect some of your organs, for example, your skull protects your brain. **Ligaments** hold the bones together yet allow movement at **joints**. The ball and socket joints at the shoulder and hip allow your limbs to move in several directions. The hinge joints at your elbow and knee let your arms and legs move up and down only. People who suffer from a disease called **arthritis** have painful joints.

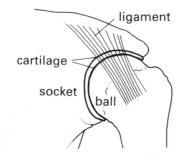

Ball and socket joint at the shoulder.

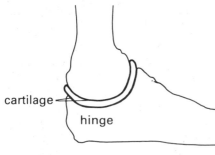

Hinge joint at the elbow.

Main bones of the skeleton.

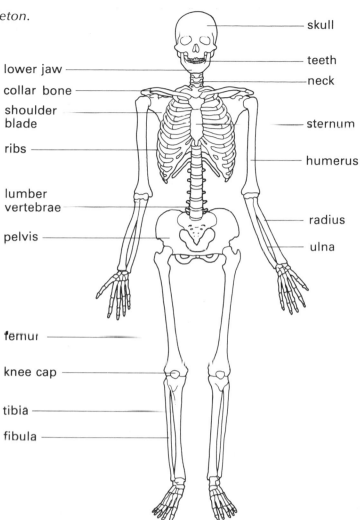

- skull
- teeth
- neck
- lower jaw
- collar bone
- shoulder blade
- sternum
- ribs
- humerus
- lumber vertebrae
- radius
- pelvis
- ulna
- femur
- knee cap
- tibia
- fibula

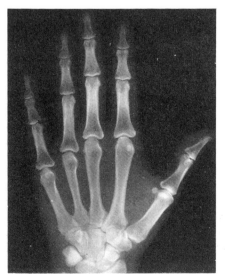

X-ray of healthy hand.

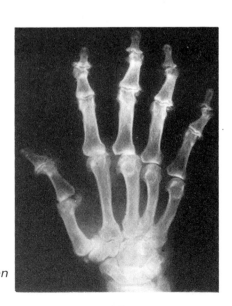

X-ray of hand of arthritis sufferer, showing swollen joints.

About half of your body weight is made up of **muscle**. If it isn't you are too fat! Each muscle is made up of millions of muscle cells which become shorter when they contract.

Try clenching your fist and watch the structures on the back of your hand move. Move your lower arm up and down and feel the muscles of your upper arm. The structures you see moving on your hand are **tendons** — they join muscles to bones. When these muscles contract they pull the bones to which they are attached together.

The muscles which move your limbs work in pairs. When one muscle contracts the other muscle of the pair relaxes. For example, when the biceps muscle contracts, the triceps muscle relaxes and the forearm moves upwards. To move the forearm downwards the biceps muscle relaxes and the triceps muscle contracts.

The skeletal system is very strong and enables us to carry out strenuous activities. It is important though that we should take great care with our bones and muscles.

Dangers of lifting

You should not attempt to lift a load which could cause you to damage your back. Over 50 000 people in Britain lose at least a day's work each year due to backache.

When you lift a load you can easily damage your back so it's worth learning how to lift correctly:

- stand close to the object
- bend your knees and keep your backbone straight
- grasp hold of the object and check you are going to be able to lift it
- straighten your knees and keep your back straight.

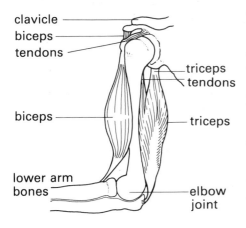

Muscles and bones of the arm.

clavicle
biceps
tendons
triceps
tendons
biceps
triceps
lower arm bones
elbow joint

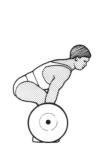 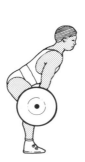 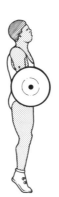 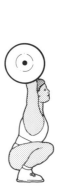 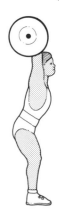

Notice how a weightlifter bends his knees to lift and keeps his back straight at all times.

If you don't bend your knees then your back muscles have to pull up the load. This strain can injure your back which may then take a long time to heal.

Sometimes you can strain your back by what is called **bad posture**. This results from sitting or standing at awkward angles. You should aim to make your back as straight as possible and sit properly in a chair. If you slouch in a chair then your back and your chest will be distorted. This may prevent you from being able to digest your food correctly and then you will suffer from indigestion and pain.

1 What are the two main functions of bones?
2 What holds bones together?
3 What joins muscles to bones?
4 Name two types of joint.
5 What parts of the body are affected by arthritis?
6 How should you lift a heavy load?
7 Describe how you should sit on a chair.
8 Why is it important to have good posture?

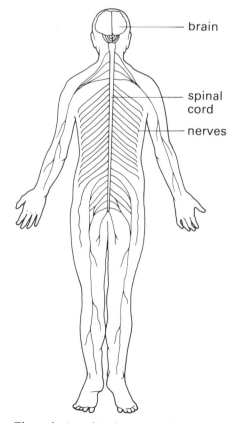

The relationship between brain, spinal cord and nerves.

The nervous system

What's happening around you?

Your eyes, ears, mouth, nose and skin contain **sense cells** which constantly detect changes going on around you and send information to your brain which decides what to do with the information.

Your **brain** and **spinal cord** make up the **central nervous system** which is linked to all parts of your body by a network of **nerves**. Each nerve is made up of bundles of long nerve cells (look back to page 7). The nerve cells carry information as nerve **impulses**.

Nerve impulses begin at sense cells and then travel along **sensory nerves** to the brain or spinal cord.

The brain is made up of about 10 000 million nerve cells which control:

- thinking, reasoning and memory
- movement, balance and reflex actions
- heart beat, respiration and body temperature.

The spinal cord, which runs through the backbone, links the brain with the rest of the body.

Main regions of the brain and their functions.

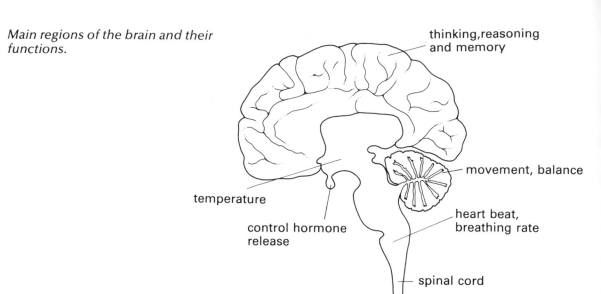

thinking, reasoning and memory

movement, balance

temperature

heart beat, breathing rate

control hormone release

spinal cord

Nerves called **motor nerves** carry impulses *from* the brain or spinal cord to muscles which respond by contracting. This system of:

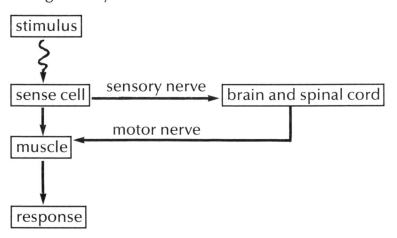

stimulus

sense cell — sensory nerve → brain and spinal cord

muscle ← motor nerve

response

keeps your body aware of what is going on and causes the correct response so that you remain fit and healthy.

Reflex actions

Reflexes are fast, automatic responses made by your body which protect you from harm. They are the result of nerve impulses passing information from sense cells to muscles at a very fast speed. For example, blinking your eyelid when an object is about to enter your eye, or removing your hand from a bowl of boiling water:

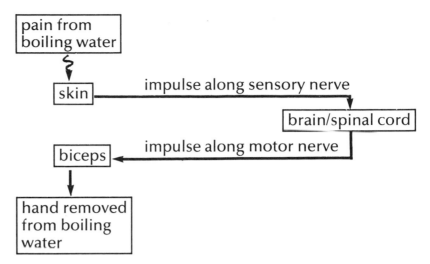

Movement of information from stimulus to response.

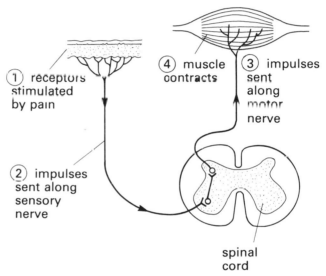

How do you see?

You see objects and people because light is reflected from them and is detected by special sense cells in your **eyes**. Light enters your eye through the transparent outer layer called the cornea. It then passes through the

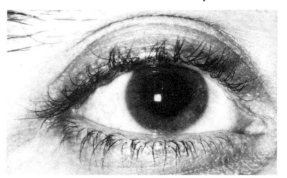

Look closely at the different parts of the eye.

pupil. This is a hole in the centre of the coloured part of the eye called the iris. The light is focused by the lens and ciliary muscles onto sense cells in the retina at the back of the eye.

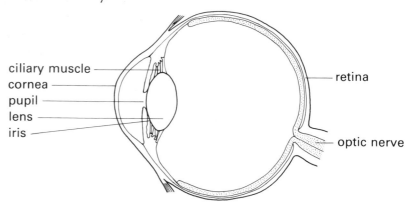

The lens of the eye focuses light on to the retina.

Sense cells called rods enable us to see objects when the light intensity is very low, e.g. at dusk and in darkness. These give us 'black and white' vision. Other sense cells called cones enable us to see in colour in high light intensities. Rods and cones convert light into tiny electrical impulses which pass to the brain along the **optic nerve**.

How do you hear?

You hear sounds because sound waves enter the ear tube and cause the ear drum to vibrate. These vibrations pass to three small bones which cause fluid in the inner ear to vibrate. The fluid is in contact with sense cells in

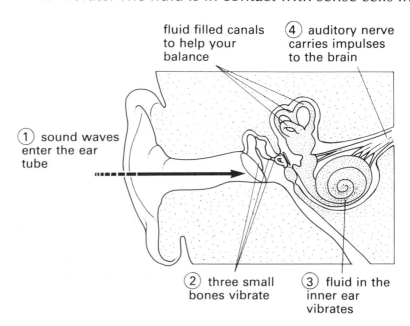

Follow through the route of the vibrations caused by sound waves.

the ear which set up electrical impulses which pass to the brain along the **auditory nerve**.

1 Name three sense organs which send information to the brain.
2 What is the function of nerves?
3 Sensory neurones carry messages to the brain. What is the purpose of motor neurones?
4 What are the main functions of the brain?
5 Draw a simple diagram to show a reflex arc.
6 What is the purpose of reflex actions?
7 What is the function of the lens in the eye?
8 Which nerve carries impulses from the ear to the brain?

The excretory system

How do you get rid of waste?

Every cell in your body produces unwanted chemical substances which must be removed from the body so that they do not poison your cells. For example, when cells release energy from food the gas **carbon dioxide** is produced; when cells in the liver break down protein an unwanted chemical substance called **urea** is produced.

Carbon dioxide is removed by the **lungs**, and the urea is removed (excreted) by the **kidneys**. Urea is stored in the form of **urine** in the **bladder** before it leaves the body. The amount of urine you produce depends on how much liquid you have drunk and how much sweat you have produced.

Sweating helps you to lose some water and salts and a small amount of urea. On a hot day you lose more sweat than on a cold day because sweating helps you to cool down.

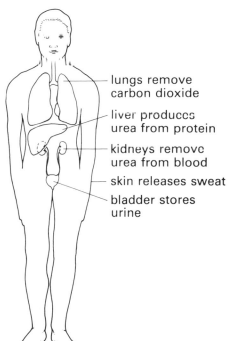

lungs remove carbon dioxide

liver produces urea from protein

kidneys remove urea from blood

skin releases sweat

bladder stores urine

Your lungs, kidneys, liver and skin get rid of unwanted chemical substances made by your body.

1 What is the waste product formed when your cells break down food and release energy?
2 Where is urea produced?
3 Where is urea removed from the blood?
4 What conditions affect the amount of urine which you produce?
5 How else does your body lose water apart from in urine?

The reproductive system

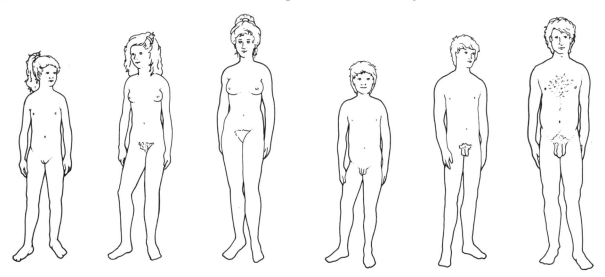

The changes that occur as a girl and boy grow up.

How do you produce children?

When you are between ten and sixteen years of age your sex organs begin to develop and the shape of your body begins to change. These changes are most noticeable in girls when their breasts develop and when they begin to have periods. Every month, blood and unwanted cells from the lining of the womb (uterus) are released through the vagina. This is called **menstruation**.

About 10–14 days after the start of each period an egg is released from an ovary. This is called **ovulation**. It is during this time that a baby can be formed if the egg joins with a sperm.

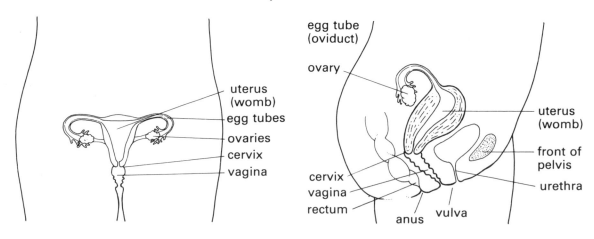

These diagrams show the reproductive system of a woman. Follow the route taken by an egg from the ovary.

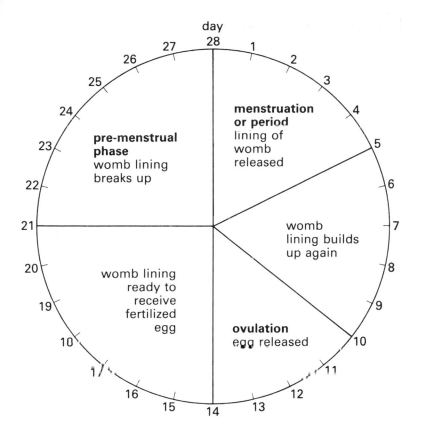

day

27 28 1

26 2

25 3

24 4

menstruation or period
lining of womb released

23 5

22 6

pre-menstrual phase
womb lining breaks up

21 7

womb lining builds up again

20 8

19 9

womb lining ready to receive fertilized egg

18 10

ovulation
egg released

17 11

16 12

15 13 14

Pregnancy can occur at any time but is more likely between the 10th and 14th day after the period starts.

Sperm are produced in the testes (*singular* testis) of the male — about 3 or 4 million sperm cells are produced each day. They flow along the sperm duct in a fluid called semen which eventually leaves the penis through a tube called the urethra. The urethra carries both urine and sperm but, of course, at different times.

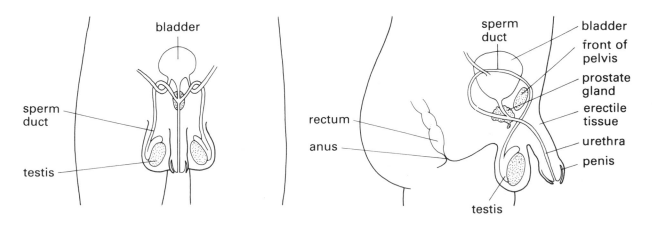

bladder

sperm duct

testis

sperm duct

bladder

front of pelvis

prostate gland

erectile tissue

urethra

penis

rectum

anus

testis

These diagrams show the reproductive system of a man. Follow the route taken by a sperm released from the testis.

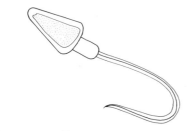

A sperm cell (×200).

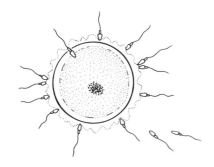

Only one sperm enters the egg and fertilizes it.

When a man and woman have **sexual intercourse** the man's penis becomes hard and erect. It is inserted into the woman's vagina which has become moist so that the penis slides in easily. The man moves his penis up and down inside the woman's vagina until he ejaculates (squirts) the semen into the vagina. The sperm then swim up into the womb and along the egg tube (oviduct) but many die on the way.

One sperm may enter the egg and this is called **fertilization**.

The fertilized egg then begins dividing and growing into many cells. These cells form an **embryo** which will develop into a baby in the thick lining of the womb. The embryo grows a heart and brain and after a few weeks is called a **fetus**. The fetus is linked to the mother by the umbilical cord attached to the placenta. Food and oxygen pass from the mother's blood through the placenta and umbilical cord and into the blood of the fetus. Waste substances such as carbon dioxide and urea are removed from the blood of the fetus and pass back into the mother's blood in the opposite direction.

The placenta cannot prevent viruses entering the baby's blood. If the mother has a disease called German measles, caused by a virus, in the first three months of pregnancy, the fetus can be severely affected.

Drugs such as heroin, nicotine in cigarettes and alcohol can also affect the growth of the fetus. It is very unwise to smoke during pregnancy.

About nine months after fertilization the baby is born.

The fetus grows and develops inside the womb.

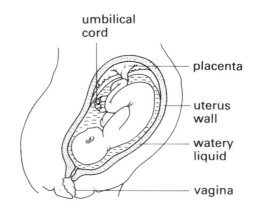

umbilical cord

placenta

uterus wall

watery liquid

vagina

1 Describe two changes which happen at puberty to (i) girls, and (ii) boys.
2 What is a 'period'?
3 How is menstruation different to ovulation?
4 Where are the sperm made?
5 What is semen?
6 Why are so many sperm produced?
7 What is fertilization?
8 Describe what happens to an egg after it has been fertilized.
9 What is the placenta?
10 Name two substances which pass from the mother to the baby through the placenta.
11 Why is it important that pregnant women do not smoke or drink alcohol?

Unit 2 | Keeping the Body Healthy

What do you eat?

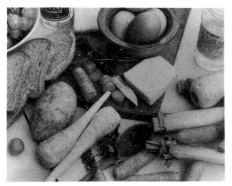

You need a variety of food for a healthy balanced diet.

The food that you eat makes up your **diet**. Each day you need to eat a variety of foods so that you eat all the different things which are essential to your health. This is called a **balanced diet** and it should contain starch, sugars, protein, fats, mineral salts (like iron and calcium), vitamins, fibre (roughage) and water. If you ate just bread or rice and nothing else you would soon be ill. Eating different foods ensures that you get all the nutrients that you need, but you also need to make sure that you have the right amount of each.

The chart on the next page shows the main sources of each nutrient of a balanced diet and why it is necessary.

You cannot tell by looking at a food what nutrients it contains. To work out whether or not you are eating a balanced diet you need to write down a list of everything you eat in one day. You will then need to look up information from food charts and find out the type of nutrients and the amount in each of the foods that you have eaten.

One of the most important things for you to think about is the amount of energy-rich food that you need to take in and the amount of energy that you use up. People who are gaining weight are taking in more energy-rich food than they need. People who are losing weight are not getting enough energy-rich food.

An average 15-year-old girl needs about 10 400 kilojoules of energy each day whereas an average 15-year-old boy needs about 12 100 kilojoules of energy each day.

Some people have to eat different food for very good reasons. These may be related to customs and religions, e.g. Jews do not eat pork, Hindus do not eat beef. Some people eat different food for medical reasons. For example, a person who is diabetic may need a diet which is free from sugar whereas someone who has heart disease may have to eat a low-fat, salt-free diet.

There is an old Chinese proverb which says 'You are what you eat'. If you wish to remain healthy you must take responsibility for what you eat.

A balanced diet provides these nutrients.

Nutrient	Source	Uses in the body
Starch	Bread, potatoes, rice	Provide you with energy for your cells to work.
Sugars	Sugar, jam, sweets, fruit	
Protein	Meat, cheese, beans	Makes all the living cells in your body.
Fats	Butter, lard, cheese	Provide energy and protect the body.
Mineral salts		
Iron	Liver, red meat	Red blood cells need iron for haemoglobin.
Calcium	Bread, cheese, milk	For strong teeth and bones.
Sodium	Salt, butter	For nerves and muscles.
Vitamins		
A	Margarine, carrots, liver	For healthy skin and good vision in dim light.
B	Meats, cereals, vegetables	To help you make use of the energy in food.
C	Fruit and vegetables	For healthy cells.
D	Milk, fatty fish, margarine	For strong bones and teeth.
Fibre (rough-age)	Wholemeal bread	To help in the removal of undigested food from the body.
Water	Almost all food	All the chemical processes which take place in your body need water. Your body is about 75% water.

1 What types of food should you eat for a 'balanced diet'?
2 Name a good source of protein.
3 Why do you need to eat food containing iron?
4 Which vitamin is required for good vision in dim light?
5 Why do you think, in general, girls and boys of the same age require different amounts of energy?
6 What type of person needs to eat a sugar-free diet?

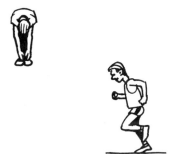

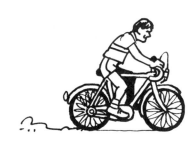

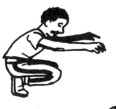

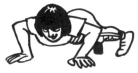

Try some of these exercises!

What's all this about exercise?

You can think of exercise as some type of movement of your body which you do for a period of time. You may move all or only a part of your body.

Why exercise?

There are four basic reasons why you may want to exercise your body.

1. General health:

   Shining hair, a clear skin, a supple co-ordinated body, greater stamina, better digestion and reduced risk of heart disease are some of the health benefits of regular exercise.

2. Heart and lungs:

   Regular exercise increases the efficiency of the heart and lung muscles as the more a muscle is used the bigger it becomes. The muscles which increase the size of the chest during breathing also become more efficient. Your heart and lungs are able then to respond quickly to a sudden change which requires greater exertion.

3. Joints:

   Exercise helps to keep your joints supple and prevent stiffness.

4. Muscles:

   Exercise increases the strength, size and efficiency of the muscles in your arms and legs.

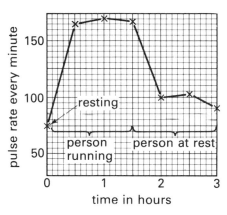

Look what happens to your pulse rate when you exercise.

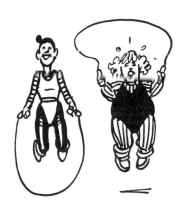

Which one are you?

What happens during exercise?

During any physical activity the cells of your body need more food and oxygen so that they can obtain the energy they need.

The heart has to pump the blood more quickly through the body so that oxygen and food get to the cells as fast as they can. The rate of breathing has to increase too so that more oxygen is breathed in and carbon dioxide is got rid of quickly.

What type of exercise should you do and how often?

Stamina exercise	20 minutes, 3 times/week	Jogging, swimming cycling, walking
Loosening-up exercise	5 minutes/day	Arm swinging, knee bending, disco dancing
Strengthening exercise	20 minutes, 3 times/week	Press-ups, sit-ups knee bends

1 How does exercise affect your heart and lungs?
2 How can you increase the size and strength of your muscles?
3 What two things are needed by your cells during exercise?
4 List two exercises which are 'stamina' exercises.
5 What type of exercise are press-ups?

Why don't you have a rest?

When you feel physically tired or fatigued you need to rest your body. Resting gives your cells a chance to repair themselves and enables your whole body to recover from stresses and strains. The most usual form of resting is sleep. If you don't have enough sleep you become tired, irritable and confused.

You usually need about 8 hours sleep per night in order to rest your brain, sense organs and muscles. Young children usually require more sleep than this because they are more active when they are awake. Sometimes you may find it difficult to go to sleep. A warm bath or hot bedtime drink can sometimes help you to sleep.

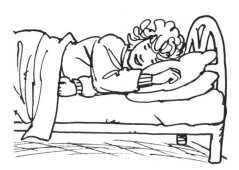

You should sleep for about 8 hours each night to relax and rest your body.

Relaxing each muscle in your body and making sure you are warm and comfortable can also help you to sleep easily.

During the working day people usually take a mid-morning and mid-afternoon break, as well as a lunch break. If they did not have a break from work they might find their concentration wandering from the task in hand, and be more likely to make errors in their work. Other forms of rest are **relaxation** and **meditation**.

We all need to have a mental and physical break from routine work. Most people find that another interest, such as a sport or hobby is a good way of relaxing. Fishing, gardening, dancing, playing football and reading are all examples of popular hobbies.

If you don't have a hobby or interest at the moment you could find out what leisure facilities are available in the area where you live. The local library usually has a list of clubs and meetings. Now is the time to try out a new hobby or learn a new skill.

Sometimes people can relax just by sitting quietly and breathing slowly. It can help to think of a very peaceful scene such as a lake or to look at a candle flame. Sometimes people learn a more thorough form of relaxation by joining a group of people who practise yoga.

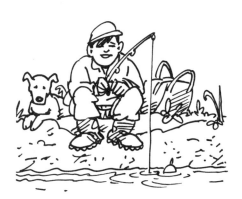

You can usually relax by being involved in a hobby or some type of activity.

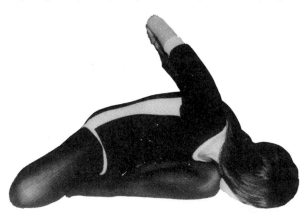

1 Why is it important to rest your body?
2 Why is it important to have a mid-morning break at work?
3 List three hobbies which you do now or have done in the past.
4 What advice could you give to someone who finds it difficult to get to sleep at night?

Preventive medicine

Medical science has made many advances in the last twenty years, but although there are many cures for diseases it is better not to become ill in the first place.

How can you stop yourself getting ill?

To keep generally healthy you must eat a balanced diet as described on pages 30 and 31. Your diet should include plenty of vitamins and minerals as your body needs these in order to resist infection. Too much sugar and fat should be avoided as they can cause problems for the heart and blood vessels as described on page 17. Plenty of rest and exercise also make you feel healthy and look healthy.

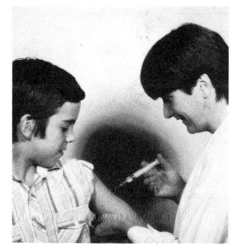

Everyone needs to be vaccinated at an early age.

To protect yourself against getting a particular disease you can be **immunized**. When you are immunized a tiny amount of a weakened form of the bacteria or virus which causes a particular disease is injected into your body. This is called **vaccine**, and the injection is called a **vaccination**. It is almost painless and is over in a few seconds.

The bacteria or viruses are too weak to cause the disease. The white blood cells in your body respond to the vaccine. They produce chemicals called **antibodies** which destroy the bacteria or viruses that have been injected. The antibodies stay in your blood for a long time and give you a built-in **resistance** to that particular disease.

How should you take care of your teeth?

You should take responsibility for looking after your own teeth. When you eat, the surface of your teeth becomes covered with a layer of sugars in which harmful bacteria grow and multiply. This layer is called **plaque**. The bacteria produce substances which will rot your teeth and infect your gums. To avoid this you should brush your teeth regularly, particularly after meals. You should use **toothpaste** and a good soft **toothbrush**, and brush gently away from your gums starting from the base of your teeth to remove food on and between the teeth. Sometimes it also helps to swill your mouth out with clear water to remove any particles of food.

Your toothbrush should be replaced when the bristles begin to flatten, as brushing your teeth with a worn toothbrush can damage your gums and fail to remove food particles from the teeth. There is a wide choice of toothpastes available which all contain an abrasive which helps to scrub the teeth. Most toothpastes also contain **fluoride** because medical evidence suggests that fluoride prevents tooth decay. In some areas fluoride is added to drinking water, and where it is not, many parents give their children fluoride tablets. **Dental floss**, which is a kind of waxy string, should also be used to clean in between teeth where particles of meat, cereals and fruit skins can become wedged.

Finally, you should visit your dentist every six months to check that your teeth are free from decay. If your dentist can stop the decay quickly, your teeth will last much longer. It is a lot cheaper to clean your teeth than to pay your dentist for fillings, caps and false teeth!

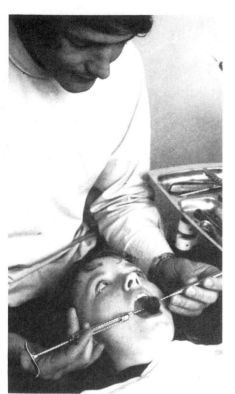

Regular visits to the dentist will help to keep your teeth and gums healthy.

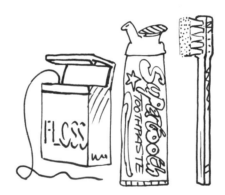

How should you look after your eyes?

Whenever you read or carry out any work you should always have good lighting because working in dim light can cause **eyestrain**. Likewise, watching television in a dark room is bad for your eyesight. Every two years you should visit an optician and have a check on your eyesight. If, in between checks, you suffer from a lot of headaches or blurred vision you should visit an optician immediately.

As you get older your eyesight may change and glasses or contact lenses may be required to help to correct your vision.

1 How can you prevent yourself getting a disease?
2 What happens when you are immunized?
3 Which cells in your blood produce antibodies?
4 What is the effect of the antibodies on the germs causing disease?
5 Why do you sometimes need a booster injection?
6 Which diseases have you been immunized against?
7 Why are girls immunized against German measles?
8 There are now many children who have not been vaccinated against whooping cough. What could happen if there was an outbreak of whooping cough?
9 Why should you brush your teeth afer meals?
10 What is dental floss?
11 Why should you visit the optician every two years?

What should you do if you think you are ill?

If you think you are ill you should visit your doctor who will ask you to describe your **symptoms**, for example headaches, pains, sickness, etc. The doctor will also examine your body for **signs** of illness, such as a rash or swellings. On the basis of these signs and symptoms the doctor may prescribe a treatment for you. It is very important that you take any medicine exactly as stated by your doctor.

It is also important that you keep your medicine away from children.

Sometimes a doctor may send you to a hospital for a check-up by a specialist, if he or she is unsure of what is wrong. This may involve something quite simple like an X-ray of a joint or the chest, or something more complex such as a series of tests on blood and urine samples.

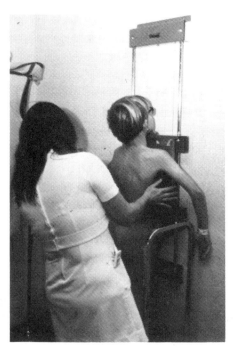

A chest X-ray can check that your lungs are free from infection.

Personal hygiene

You should be responsible for your own health and for the health of the people you share a house with. Your personal habits and **hygiene** (keeping clean) are very important in reducing the spread of disease. There are some families who are always suffering from 'tummy bugs' usually because they don't realize the importance of hygiene. Very often the 'bugs' causing the disease are passed on because they don't wash their hands when they have been to the toilet. In a school it is very easy for a 'bug' to be passed round if you don't wash your hands after visiting the toilet. Many diseases throughout the world such as typhoid, cholera, bilharzia and dysentery are spread because contaminated faeces get into drinking water.

You should wash your hands after every time you visit the toilet.

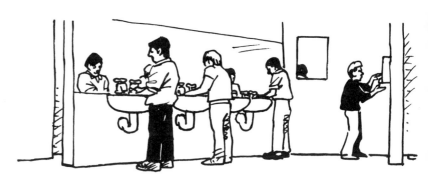

What should you do to keep yourself clean?

Hands

Almost everything you touch is covered in bacteria and viruses. If you have germs on your hands when you eat, these germs get into your body and cause you to become ill with an upset tummy, sickness and diarrhoea. So you should:

- always wash your hands before eating, or before preparing food
- always wash your hands after visiting the toilet
- don't wash your hands only when they look or feel dirty.

Feet

Most people often spend time looking after their hands but ignore the cleanliness of their feet. You should:

Take as much care of your feet as the rest of your body.

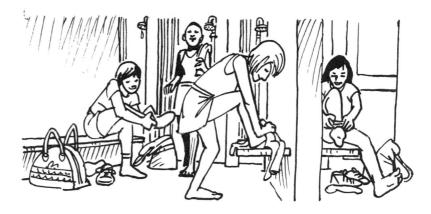

- wash your feet every day and dry them carefully
- put on a clean pair of socks or tights every day
- wear a different pair of shoes in the evening so that the shoes worn in the daytime have a chance to dry out and air
- cut your toenails straight across to keep them short and clean

If you have damp, sweaty feet and do not follow the above guidelines you may develop **athlete's foot**. This is a skin infection caused by a fungus which takes quite a long time to get rid of.

Armpits

You should wash the **sweat** away from your armpits every day because when you sweat, the bacteria on your skin start to grow. Stale sweat and bacteria soon begin to smell very unpleasant, so much so that many people now use an antiperspirant to reduce sweating, or a deodorant to help reduce the smell. It's a good idea though to wear a clean shirt or blouse every day.

Clothes made of natural or mixed fibres let your skin 'breathe' much more easily than clothes made of 100% man-made fibres such as polyester.

Genital area (crotch)

You should wash your genital area every day with warm water as this is another area of the body where sweat and bacteria collect. When you wash your genital area it is important to wash from front to back so that germs don't get spread from your anus to your sex organs.

If your penis has a foreskin you need to push the foreskin back gently to wash the top of the penis. If this is not done germs can breed under the foreskin and cause infection and sores.

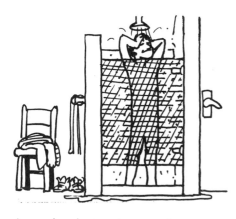

A regular shower is a good way to keep yourself clean.

It's a good idea to wear cotton or cotton/polyester underclothes as these reduce the amount of sweat which forms around your genital area and anus. Underclothes should be changed each day.

Hair

When your hair looks dull or greasy it needs to be washed so that it looks clean and shiny. Some people wash their hair every day, others twice a week or once a week. Whenever you wash your hair you should use a mild shampoo (not soap) and warm water and make sure that you rinse away the shampoo in plenty of clean water.

If you suffer from **dandruff** you will need to use a medicated shampoo to help remove all the dead skin on your scalp. If your head itches a lot you may have caught **head lice**. Surprisingly enough, head lice like clean hair. You will need to put a special lotion on your hair which your chemist or doctor will be able to supply to kill the lice.

1 Why it is important to wash your hands after visiting the toilet?
2 How can you prevent 'athlete's foot'?
3 Why is it important to wash your body every day?
4 What type of fabric or material should you wear next to your skin?
5 What action should you take if you have dandruff?
6 What advice would you give to someone who had head lice?

Unit 3

Emotional Well-being

How are you feeling?

You may be feeling happy and cheerful or miserable and fed-up. Your **emotions** are how you respond mentally to a situation. Different people respond in different ways to the same situation. For example, when watching a comedian on TV some people will giggle or laugh at the jokes while others just smile. If you are in a situation which makes you feel unhappy, you may show your feelings by either looking unhappy, or by crying.

People may also show the same emotion in different ways. For example, we may show our love for someone physically by hugging and kissing them, or emotionally by worrying and caring about them.

Young children have to learn to control their emotions. Young babies and children often cry when they cannot have what they want immediately, but as you get older you learn to control your outward show of emotion even though you may feel the emotion inside. When you cannot control your emotions you may find that you lose control over your actions. Sometimes people say 'I was so angry I just didn't know what I was doing'.

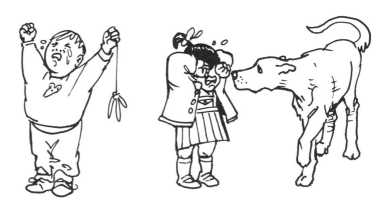

Young children often show their emotions very clearly!

Loss of control can have serious effects on other people. Sometimes a driver of a car who loses control of his or her emotions can injure or even kill another person. People sometimes hit out at another person and are sorry for their action almost immediately afterwards. If you feel angry or upset about a situation there are many ways of coping with your emotions. Sometimes it helps just to take a few deep breaths and try to relax for a minute. This gives you time to be aware that you are upset and feeling an extreme of emotion and to take control of your feelings by becoming calm. Once you have your emotion under control you may find that you are in a better position to sort out the situation that you are in.

If you find yourself worrying about a situation such as an exam or an interview, imagine the *worst* thing that could happen to you and then think about how you could handle your fears. For example, suppose you fail *all* your exams, what will you do in this situation? Thinking clearly and rationally about your worst fears can make you realise that they can be coped with. In every case of worry and anxiety it always helps to talk the problem over with someone else.

Many young people find it very difficult to talk to their parents. Sometimes you may find it easier to talk to someone you don't know very well such as the parent of a friend, or a teacher at school who you seem to get on with. It may seem awkward to talk to your doctor but if you have worries about your body the best person to confide in is your doctor. Your doctor will treat what you say in confidence. Some people who belong to a church or youth group often find there the kind of person they can talk to.

Have you ever thought that you may be the type of person who someone else can talk to? In this situation it is best not to offer advice to your friends but to help them to work out their own answers.

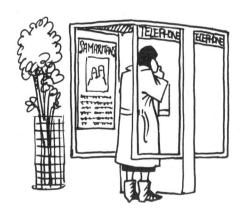

For people who feel that there is no one that they can talk to or turn to for help there is usually a telephone number for the Samaritans in your phone book. The Samaritans will always listen to you talk and will give help and advice as needed.

1 Describe two outward signs of an emotional feeling.
2 Why is it important to learn to control your emotions?
3 What should you do if you find yourself worrying about a situation?
4 What type of people could you go to if you wanted to talk about your feelings?

What is stress?

Stress is difficult to describe but you may have experienced it during your life. It occurs when excessive demands are made on your body. These demands may be emotional, which may cause feelings of **depression**, or physical, which may cause headaches, 'butterflies' in your stomach, a dry mouth or a rapid heart beat.

Stress can be caused by any factor which seems to put an extra 'load' on the body, for example noise, drugs, chemicals, tiredness, infections, surgery, mental upset, emotional upset, and many other factors. If you are subjected to stress factors over a period of time you may find yourself becoming irritable, not sleeping easily, losing your concentration and becoming depressed. People who suffer from stress sometimes suffer from heart disease and stomach ulcers. Asthma and skin disorders are often thought to be related to stress.

What is a stressful situation for one person may just be a challenge to another. For example, if you run to catch a bus your heart and lungs adjust quickly to the demand for oxygen. This situation is short-lived because you either catch the bus or miss it. In either case your body can return to normal very quickly. If however, the stimulus of running for a bus was continued over a longer period of time the demands or stresses on your body would be prolonged and you might suffer from a heart attack. Athletes are able to respond to such a stimulus over a long period of time because they prepare themselves for this by careful training.

When your body is under stress, part of your nervous system is stimulated to release chemical substances called **hormones**. One of these hormones is **adrenaline** which has several effects on the body. It causes a rapid pulse, deep rapid breathing, and the diverting of blood from the skin to the muscles. All these changes make your body prepared for instant physical action.

However, problems can occur when adrenaline is released into your blood at times when your body is not involved in physical activity. This is because adrenaline causes sugar and fats to flow in the blood. If these sugars and fats are not used up by the body during physical activity they become deposited inside the arteries. These fatty deposits cause the arteries to become narrow so that less blood flows through them and this may lead to problems with your heart and circulation.

Which person is likely to be suffering from stress?

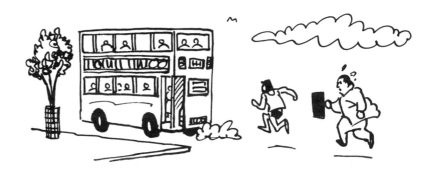

How do you cope with stress?

Your personality affects the way in which you react to a stressful situation and different people react to the same stimulus in many different ways.

When you are under stress you need to feel that you can cope with the situation you are in. Sometimes you can help yourself become calm by doing something which you find relaxing such as kicking a football, listening to music, riding a bike or doing any type of physical exercise. We all need to learn to recognize the signs of stress in ourselves. Whenever you feel your heart beating very fast and you experience headaches and tension you should learn to relax by breathing slowly and deeply so as to make yourself become calm. It often helps if you imagine a place where you can be very relaxed and think about that place for a few moments.

It can also help to talk to someone who is sympathetic such as a good friend, a parent or a teacher. Just by talking to someone you often find that you can control the situation which causes you stress. That is the first step in sorting out your problems.

How can you prevent stress?

You may find that doing some regular exercise every day will help to make you less affected by stress. Most people have a relaxing hobby or interest which gives their body a chance to 'unwind'.

---

1 Describe two symptoms of stress in your body.
2 What problems are caused by your body being affected by stress over a long period of time?
3 Describe three effects of adrenaline on your body.
4 What can you do to relax if your body is suffering from stress?

What is depression?

Depression is one of the commonest forms of mental illness. Usually, it only lasts for a few hours, then disappears but sometimes people become unhappy and distressed for long periods of time. This may cause the person to become irritable, lose their appetite, and find difficulty in sleeping. People who are depressed may feel that they cannot cope with life and their pattern of behaviour becomes far from normal.

Because everyone's pattern of behaviour is different it is sometimes difficult to decide when a person requires treatment for depression. For example, in the case of the person who becomes very upset and depressed at losing a close relative the depression is usually only temporary. If, however, the person continues to be disturbed and upset for a long period of time they may be suffering from a more severe form of depression. In some cases the person becomes very distressed and loses interest in life.

Depression can be treated medically by taking anti-depressant drugs which cause the nervous system to become more active.

In common with most illnesses it is better to avoid depression than to cure depression. This can be done by achieving a balance of work and relaxation. Problems which appear impossible to solve often sort themselves out after a period of relaxation or a change of activity or a regular break from routine.

A good balance of work and play, as well as having people to talk to, are very important in avoiding depression.

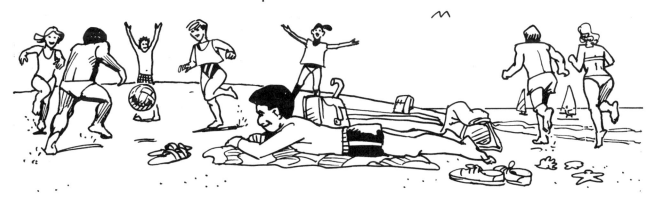

Holidays are important for relaxation and a change of routine.

1 What are the common symptoms of depression?
2 Describe two things which you could do to help avoid depression.

Death and grief

There is an old saying that, 'The only certainty in life is death', because our bodies don't last forever and they eventually wear out. The moment of dying is thought to be similar to going to sleep or becoming unconscious. Unfortunately, some people suffer illness for a long time before they die. During this time they may be able to adapt to their suffering and illness and prepare for death. Other people die suddenly, perhaps in an accident or through a sudden malfunction in their body. People who die in this way have no time to prepare for death, and their relatives are often very upset by the sudden death of someone they love and care for very deeply.

The family and friends of someone who has died need a great deal of help and support during their grief so that they can 'work through' their grief. These people are suffering from shock and need to express their feelings, usually through crying. Some people though are unable to release their feelings and this can lead to all sorts of problems. It is often helpful to encourage these people to share their grief and release their feelings. Friends and neighbours can help a person cope with grief by talking about the person who has died. On these occasions it is often helpful to show compassion to the person who is grieving and this may involve some form of physical contact, for example, holding hands or putting your arm around someone to comfort them.

When a person has released their feelings of grief, they often become angry and ask 'Why has this happened?' To prevent this it is important that people should realise that death is inevitable and other people who have suffered the loss of a loved one have been able to cope with death in their lives. It is important that you show sympathy and understanding to people who are grieving.

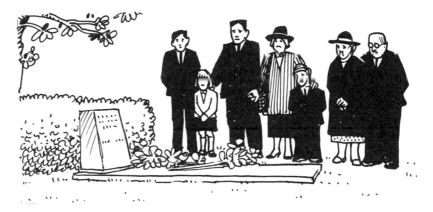

Many people find peace of mind and comfort from their faith and religious beliefs which helps them to accept the inevitability of death and the certainty of life after death.

1 Why is it often important for someone who has lost a close relative or friend to talk about their loss?
2 Why is it sometimes important for someone to cry after losing a close relative or friend?
3 How can you help a person who is suffering from grief?

Unit 4

Problems and Treatment

What are drugs?

Drugs are chemical substances which affect either your tissues and organs or affect the viruses and bacteria living inside your body. They are usually taken for medical reasons but some people take certain drugs, for example heroin, in order to obtain pleasurable sensations. In many cases this leads to the person becoming addicted to a particular drug which can have serious effects on their health. In general though, drugs can be very useful to most people and many lives have been saved by the correct use of drugs.

Drugs affect different people in different ways and sometimes they can cause side-effects, for example, headache, feeling sick or dizzy, or suffering an allergic reaction such as a skin rash.

In society today many people take drugs for minor problems, because they mistakenly think that drugs will help to solve their problems. They do not do this. Instead drugs only temporarily remove the symptoms of the problem and not the cause. For example, if you cannot sleep due to anxiety or some special problem, then it is better to find a solution to the problem, rather than take sleeping tablets. Likewise, if you have a headache, an aspirin may 'cure' your headache, but the cause of the headache may still be present. If nothing is done about the cause of the headache it will keep recurring and may be a symptom of something more serious. Therefore it is better to find out the cause of the headache than to continually blot out the pain.

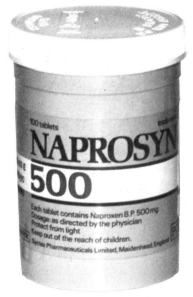

Taking tablets can help relieve the symptoms but don't always remove the problem.

Table showing the most commonly prescribed drugs.

Numbers of prescriptions (UK/year)	Type of drug
10 million	Stimulants
17 million	Sleeping pills
18 million	Painkillers
19 million	Tranquillizers
7.5 million	Anti-depressants

Prescribed drugs

Certain drugs are essential in order to maintain good health in some people. For example, you may know of someone with **diabetes**. Diabetics are people who are unable to control the amount of sugar in their blood because they cannot produce enough insulin. Therefore they need a regular injection of **insulin** to keep them alive. The numbers of people suffering from diabetes has increased rapidly during the last 35 years, possibly due to the increase in the amount of sugar in our daily diet. There are many other drugs which doctors are now able to give to patients which help them to lead longer, active lives. As medical science makes new discoveries so pain and suffering is reduced.

Non-prescribed drugs – nicotine and alcohol

One of the most widely used drugs which does not require a doctor's prescription is **nicotine**, which is an **addictive** drug found in cigarettes. When you smoke, the nicotine is absorbed into your blood stream and has a relaxing effect on the body. People who become addicted to nicotine need to smoke more and more to produce the same effect on their body. Unfortunately many children in their early teens become nicotine addicts and this can have a very dangerous effect on their health.

Women who smoke cigarettes when they are pregnant may give birth to babies that have not developed normally or fully.

Another commonly used drug is **alcohol** which is a chemical found in beers, wines and spirits. Alcohol slows down your reactions and causes a lack of co-ordination of muscles. People drink alcohol because it usually makes them feel more relaxed and able to talk to other people more easily. An occasional alcoholic drink may not cause any harm, but several drinks each day can lead to serious problems. One of the effects of drinking alcohol for a period of years can be a diseased liver, an ulcerated stomach, weak heart muscles, cancer of the mouth, high blood pressure and depression.

Women who drink excessively when they are pregnant run the risk of the alcohol affecting their baby. In particular, it can slow down the rate of development of the baby.

Alcohol can also affect our ability to think clearly and quickly. This is a particular problem to motorists and is a major source of road accidents. No one should drink and drive as even one drink can make you react more slowly in an emergency situation.

In Britain there are strict controls on drinking and driving, and anyone found driving a car or motorcycle with over 80 milligrams of alcohol in their blood will be prosecuted. See Unit 14.

---

1 What is a drug?
2 Describe some side-effects of taking drugs.
3 What is an alternative to taking a sleeping pill if you cannot sleep?
4 What should you do if you keep having headaches?
5 What drug is needed by diabetics to help them control the sugar in their blood?
6 What addictive drug is found in cigarettes?
7 What is the effect of alcohol on your body?
8 What are some of the long-term effects of drinking alcohol?
9 Why should a pregnant woman drink less alcohol?

What other drugs can be addictive?

When we read in the newspapers about the 'drug problem', 'drug-taking', 'addicts' and 'pushers', it is usually **illegal drugs** which are being referred to. These fall into one of the categories shown below.

Type of drug	Drug	Uses and effects	Characteristics
Narcotics	Morphine	Pain reliever.	Addictive.
	Heroin	Feeling of well-being, euphoria.	Addictive, more is needed each time to experience the same effect.
Hallucinogens	LSD ('acid')	Hallucinations or 'trips'.	Causes abnormal behaviour and accidents.
	Cannabis ('dope', 'grass', 'hashish', 'pot')	Hallucinations, feeling of well-being.	If it becomes addictive it can cause mental and physical breakdown.
Barbiturates		Sedatives, depress normal function of brain.	Addictive, interact with alcohol.
Amphetamines		Stimulate central nervous system, increase ability to stay awake.	After-effect of depression and exhaustion, increase in aggression, and irritability, addictive.

The use of any of the drugs in the table without a prescription is illegal and anyone found in possession of them will be charged with a criminal offence.

Morphine is used medically to relieve pain whereas heroin, when injected into the blood stream, produces a feeling of well-being. Users of heroin can quickly become addicted to the drug. When this happens the body needs more and more heroin to produce the same effect. This is the great danger of drug addiction.

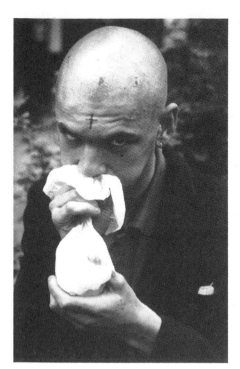

What are the dangers of glue-sniffing?

Many glues and other household products contain a chemical **solvent** which stops them going solid. Glue-sniffing is sometimes referred to as **solvent abuse** because people breathe in the fumes given off by the solvent.

The fumes affect the brain and produce a temporary pleasant sensation. In some people though this quickly leads to delirium and unconsciousness and when affected in this way many people have died as a result of falling down stairs or into water, or from choking on their own vomit. Glue-sniffers often have a cough, sore eyes, sores around the mouth and they are irritable and moody. If you know anyone who is a glue-sniffer, they desperately need help and advice. It is a very dangerous habit and can become addictive.

What are the effects of addiction?

There are many dangers associated with using illegal drugs, especially those drugs which are injected into the blood. Firstly, there is no control over the quality of the drug and impurities may be present which can cause serious side-effects. Secondly, the strength of the drug is unknown so it is difficult to control the amount of drug being injected. Thirdly, injecting with unsterilized needles can cause other diseases such as blood poisoning, hepatitis and AIDS.

AIDS is thought to be caused by a virus called the HIV virus (Human Immune Deficiency Virus). The danger of contracting HIV is one of the more serious effects of misusing drugs. If you inject yourself with a needle and syringe which has been used by someone else you are at risk. If it was used by someone carrying the HIV virus you could be injecting the virus into your blood.

People who are addicted to non-prescribed drugs are often unable to have a regular job and do not have the money to pay for their drugs. Some drug addicts may become 'pushers' (people who sell drugs to others) and in this way they make enough money to buy their own drugs. Some drug addicts may steal money from friends and family in order to pay for drugs. These people need help and this is available but addicts must first of all admit that they have a serious drug problem and visit a doctor or a clinic where they can be prescribed drugs

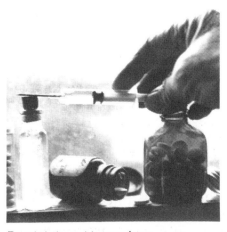

Don't inject. Never share.

whose strength and purity is carefully controlled. Regular visits to a clinic for counselling and group therapy can be successful in helping an addict to stop taking drugs.

During this time these people need a great deal of support and help from their family and friends.

---

1 What type of drugs are morphine and heroin?
2 What is meant by the term 'an addictive drug'?
3 Why is it harmful to your body to take cannabis?
4 Some people take amphetamines to stay awake. What are some of the after-effects on the body of amphetamines?
5 Why is it very dangerous to use illegal drugs?
6 Describe three health problems caused by glue-sniffing or solvent abuse.
7 What advice could you give to someone who was addicted to drugs?

What are the causes of disorders and handicaps?

If you are fit and healthy it is very difficult to imagine what it must be like to be a handicapped person. Trying to lead a normal life presents handicapped people with a number of difficulties which they have to overcome, in addition to the everyday problems that we all face.

Sometimes babies are born handicapped, but people can become handicapped or disabled at any time during their life.

There are two types of handicap, physical and mental.

Physical handicap

There are over three million physically handicapped people in the United Kingdom. These are people who do not have the full use of one or more limbs or who are unable to see or hear fully. In the majority of cases these people have no form of mental handicap.

A number of people are handicapped from birth as a result of a **congenital defect**. Such defects can arise as a result of the mother having suffered from an illness such as German measles during pregnancy. In other cases drugs taken by the mother during pregnancy may affect the developing baby. About 30 years ago a drug called **thalidomide**, which was taken by women to prevent early morning sickness, caused many children to be born blind or deaf or with one or more limbs missing or deformed.

A number of children are born each year with physical defects caused by problems which arise during development of the fetus. These are called **genetic defects** (hereditary defects). Cystic fibrosis, which causes problems to the respiratory and digestive systems is a genetic disease.

Many more people become handicapped each year as a result of accidents which can happen at any time and at any place. In addition, diseases such as polio and multiple sclerosis can severely affect the use of limbs and heart attacks and strokes can also cause disablement at any time.

Sometimes young children can accidentally become mentally or physically handicapped when they are immunized against certain diseases. In the case of whooping cough vaccination there is a very slight risk that the child may suffer disablement.

In all cases of accidental disability, people have to adjust to a completely different way of life. They may be unable to continue with their job or normal schooling, and possibly have to move home in order to have both easier access to their house and mobility within it.

How do people cope with physical handicaps?

Most people who are physically handicapped would like to be able to go shopping, to go to the cinema, to be able to work in a normal office and to live in a normal house. In the past this was not possible because most buildings did not have easy access for a wheelchair, as many buildings had steps, narrow doors and inadequate toilet facilities. Nowadays, new buildings in towns and cities are designed to take wheelchairs and special toilet facilities are provided. The homes of handicapped people can have doors and worktops altered so that the handicapped person can be independent of other people. Many handicapped people now have specially modified cars so that they are mobile and it is becoming increasingly possible for a physically handicapped

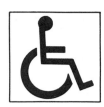

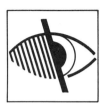

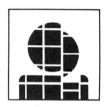

Can you work out what each of the signs mean?

Blind or partially sighted
Mentally handicapped
Deaf or hard of hearing
Physically handicapped

person to lead as full a life as someone who has use of all their limbs and organs.

Blind and partially sighted

Someone goes blind in the United Kingdom every 45 minutes and there are over 145 000 (in 1988) registered blind or partially sighted people. The National Health Service provides treatment and help for blind and partially sighted people but the Royal National Institute for the Blind is the major source of help. It provides a complete range of services including help in finding employment. Local libraries can now supply large print books or a 'talking book' service.

Deaf or hard of hearing

Over two and a half million people in the United Kingdom suffer from loss of hearing. Children are usually tested for hearing throughout their school life as early diagnosis often enables the hearing problem to be corrected. The National Health Service provides hearing aids and special schools or teachers for deaf children and the Royal National Institute for the Deaf offers help in learning to communicate by sign language and lip reading. Many television programmes nowadays have subtitles available to assist those people with hearing difficulties.

Mental handicap

One child in every hundred is born mentally handicapped and there are over half a million people with a mental handicap in the United Kingdom. Mentally handicapped people suffer from some form of brain damage which may also prevent them from controlling some of their physical actions. One of the commonest forms of mental handicap is Down's syndrome which is caused by a genetic defect resulting in the baby being born with an extra chromosome in all its cells. Tremendous advances have been made in the care of Down's syndrome sufferers and many now lead a more normal life than people would have believed possible ten years ago.

How do people cope with mental handicaps?

Mentally handicapped children usually need special care and full-time help. If parents are not able to cope with the demands of caring for a mentally handicapped child, especially if there are other children in the family, there are special residential schools with trained assistants to look after them. Even when mentally handicapped children become adult they usually have a mental age of a child and still need a great deal of care and devotion.

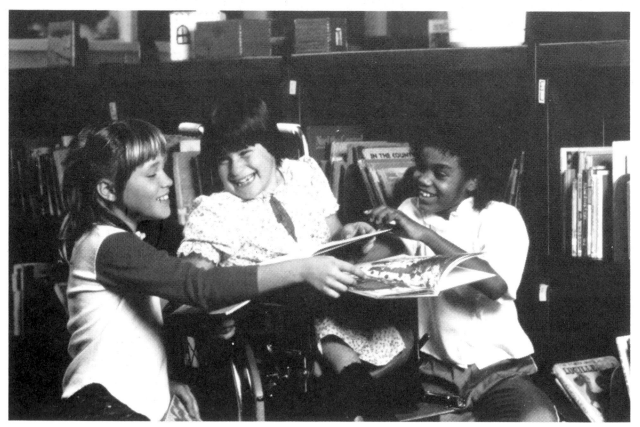

Some handicapped children go to an ordinary school and can lead an almost normal life.

1 What are the two main types of handicap?
2 What can be the effect on the baby of a mother having German measles during pregnancy?
3 Name one inherited disease which causes physical handicap.
4 Describe how an able-bodied person could become handicapped during their life.
5 What is a 'Down's syndrome' baby?
6 How can a person's home be specially adapted if the person is handicapped?
7 What help is available for someone who is (i) blind or partially sighted, or (ii) deaf or hard of hearing?

HYGIENE AND COMMUNITY HEALTH
Unit 5   Food Hygiene

Why does food go bad?

Certain tiny organisms in the air called **bacteria** and **fungi** cause food to go bad. Fungi appear as moulds on bread, cheese and fruit and make food unpleasant to eat. Bacteria grow in fish, meat and milk and make them dangerous to eat. Food can also go bad or, as we sometimes say, 'go off', without being affected by fungi or bacteria. This is because chemical substances called **enzymes**, which are present naturally in food, start to break down the food after a few days. This may make it smell unpleasant.

We need to prevent food going bad so that it can be kept for a longer time than just a few days. There are several different methods of preventing food from going bad and these are described next. Each one slows down or stops the action of the bacteria, fungi, or enzymes.

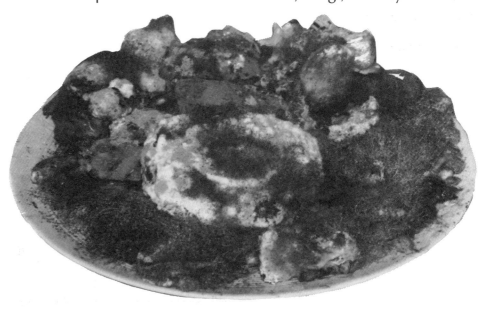

This food will keep fresh for longer, as the air has been excluded.

How do we store and preserve food?

There are many different ways of preserving food. Each method has advantages and disadvantages. Whenever possible though, you should eat food which is fresh, as this ensures that you get the most vitamins and mineral salts from your food.

Sealing and packaging

Most fresh food which you buy in a shop is covered or wrapped up to prevent air from reaching the food. The advantage of covering food in see-through polythene is that the food is kept fresh and clean. Sometimes food is **vacuum packed**. This means that all the air from around the food is removed when it is packed. Cheese, coffee and meats are often vacuum packed and you can hear a slight hiss as air goes into the packet when it is opened.

Food stores

You may have a larder, pantry or kitchen cabinet at home where you keep dry food which is in packets or tins. Dry foods such as flour, biscuits, tea, coffee and sugar are kept in these places to prevent cockroaches, mice and rats from reaching the food and to keep food away from the moist air of steamy kitchens.

Drying

Bacteria and fungi need water to grow. When food is dried (dehydrated) all the water is removed so that bacteria and fungi organisms cannot grow, e.g. dried soup, dried milk, raisins, sultanas, cake mix.

Refrigeration

Bacteria and fungi also need a warm temperature in order to grow. When you put food into a refrigerator at a temperature of about 4°C the organisms grow very slowly. Refrigeration therefore enables most foods to be kept reasonably fresh for several days. It also has the following advantages:

- the food is kept clean, cool and away from dust and insects
- left-over food can be kept for a few days until needed
- you only need to shop every few days
- meals can be cooked a day or two in advance
- foods can taste nicer if they are served chilled.

A new method of refrigeration has recently been developed which depends on the temperature of the

Refrigerated food keeps fresh for several days.

food being kept constant at 1°C, from the time the food is packed until it is bought. This lengthens the shelf life of the food and avoids many of the main disadvantages of deep freezing.

Deep freezing

Freezing food is one of the easiest and safest ways of storing food. By freezing and packing food at −18°C and then storing it just below that temperature, food can be kept for long periods of time. At these temperatures bacteria and fungi cannot grow and the activity of enzymes virtually ceases. For some foods though, the flavour and quality gradually deteriorate if stored for a long time.

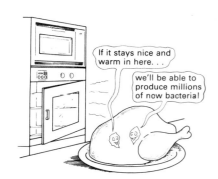

A common cause of food poisoning is partly cooked chicken.

Food which has been frozen must be defrosted or thawed properly before it is cooked. In the case of a larger joint of meat, enough time must be allowed for it to thaw through completely. If this does not happen the middle of the joint may remain frozen and not be cooked properly. Bacteria in the meat will not be destroyed by the cooking and this can cause **food poisoning**. Inadequate thawing of frozen chickens prior to cooking is quite a common cause of food poisoning.

Most types of food can be frozen but the most popular foods for freezing are usually meat, fish, vegetables, bread, ice cream and soft fruits. Strawberries and raspberries though, lose their shape and some of their taste as a result of deep freezing and this is a disadvantage.

Deep freezing has the following advantages:

- you can buy food in bulk and this reduces costs
- fruit and vegetables can be bought cheaply when in season and stored
- complete meals can be cooked in advance and stored until needed
- there is a ready source of food should friends arrive unexpectedly.

Canning

When food is being prepared for canning it is heated to a high temperature in large pressure cookers. The high temperature kills all the bacteria and fungi and destroy the enzymes. The hot food is then put into sterilized metal cans and sealed to keep the air out, e.g. soup, baked beans, sardines, ham, vegetables.

Food can be stored for a long time, in some cases for up to several years so long as the can is undamaged. If there

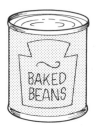 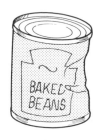

Make sure the cans you buy are not dented or rusty.

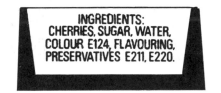

INGREDIENTS:
CHERRIES, SUGAR, WATER,
COLOUR E124, FLAVOURING,
PRESERVATIVES E211, E220.

Preservatives help to increase the shelf life of food.

is a hole in the can, air will reach the food and the bacteria and fungi in the air will make it go bad.

Sometimes the can begins to go rusty and this can destroy the metal and let air into the food. When you buy a can you should check that it is not damaged or dented. If you have a can at home that starts to bulge outwards you should throw it away. The food inside will have gone bad and be releasing gases which cause the can to expand.

Salting and smoking

Some food can be preserved by adding salt or smoking. Adding salt to food removes the water from it and in so doing prevents bacteria or fungi in the food, e.g. bacon, fish and vegetables, from growing.

Pork and fish can also be preserved by hanging it in smoke-filled rooms where chemicals in the smoke kill any bacteria or fungi present in the food.

Sugar

When fruit is made into jams or bottled, a lot of sugar is added. This removes the water from the food and from the bacteria and fungi in the food and, in doing so, kills them. Heating the fruit to make jam kills remaining bacteria and fungi.

Chemical preservatives

Many foods contain chemical preservatives which slow down the rate at which bacteria and fungi reproduce and grow, e.g. fruit juice, salad cream and liver sausage. All foods containing food preservatives are required to state which preservatives they contain and these are described in terms of an international code, e.g. some jam contains the preservative E220, sulphur dioxide.

Irradiation

In some countries, food is preserved by exposing it to radiation from radioactive chemicals. This destroys all bacteria and fungi so that the food keeps longer. Some people believe there are possible health hazards from using irradiated food and it is banned in Britain at the moment, except for patients in hospitals who need sterile food.

Irradiated food may be allowed to be sold in shops, however, in the near future, as the laws are being modified.

Pasteurization

Milk which has not been treated in any way goes sour fairly quickly due to the activity of bacteria. Almost all milk is now heated to a temperature of 71°C for about 17 seconds and then cooled very rapidly. This process is called **pasteurization** and it kills most of these harmful bacteria. Milk which has been treated in this way will keep for several days and does not lose its flavour.

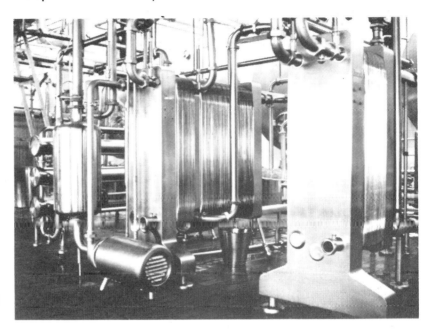

Almost all milk is heat-treated to kill the harmful bacteria.

1 Why is some food sold 'vacuum packed'?
2 What type of food should be kept in a larder or pantry?
3 List two examples of dried food.
4 Why does dried food keep for a long time?
5 What happens to bacteria and fungi when they are put into a refrigerator?
6 List three advantages of using a refrigerator.
7 Why should you defrost frozen meat thoroughly before cooking it?
8 List two disadvantages of using a freezer.
9 When food is put into cans, why is it heated to a high temperature?
10 How does smoking food help to preserve it?
11 Why is sugar added to fruit when making jam?
12 Describe how milk is pasteurized.

Unit 6 | Preparation of Food for Eating

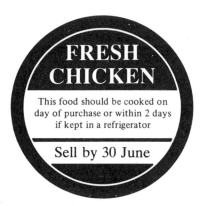

Check the 'sell by' date before you buy your food.

When you buy food in a shop there is usually a 'sell-by' date on the container. This is the date by which the shopkeeper has to sell the food. Usually food can be eaten a few days after the sell-by date, especially if it is kept in a fridge, e.g. cheese, milk, yoghurt, meat, prepared salads.

Why should you wash food before eating it?

You should always wash fruit, vegetables, meat and fish before eating or cooking them. The water washes away any dirt, bacteria, fungi, or chemical spray which may be on the food. If you are in a country where the water supply is not safe for drinking you should always wash fruit in water which has been purified with chemical tablets.

What happens to food when it is cooked?

The heat used to cook food kills bacteria and fungi. It is therefore very important that food should be thoroughly cooked so that all harmful bacteria and fungi are destroyed. All fresh food should be perfectly safe to eat but whenever you are in doubt you should cook the food. This is particularly important in the case of foods containing meat or fish. Meat pies and sausages can be a common source of food poisoning caused by a bacterium called *Salmonella*.

Cookery books and the instructions on packets or tins of food tell you how to cook different types of food. Microwave cookers are a very efficient way of ensuring

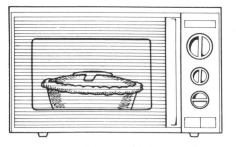

Microwaves heat food thoroughly and kill all bacteria.

that food is fully cooked and therefore safe to eat. They cook food from the inside outwards, by heating the water molecules in the food and killing all bacteria and fungi in the process. Many cafes and restaurants use microwaves to cook food, especially 'take-away' food such as pasties and pies.

What is food poisoning?

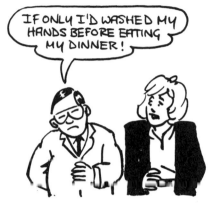

*Make sure **you** don't get food poisoning!*

If you eat food which contains certain types of bacteria you may get food poisoning. The symptoms are sickness (vomiting), pains in your muscles and diarrhoea. Food that has not been washed or which was poorly cooked before eating is the main source of food poisoning. Chicken and duck are two foods which normally contain many of the *Salmonella* bacteria responsible for food poisoning. These foods should always be cooked thoroughly, especially if they are eaten up as 'left-overs'. Food poisoning can be very dangerous to young children and elderly people and it should be treated immediately.

The following points help to prevent the outbreak of food poisoning:

- cook food thoroughly
- cover food after cooking
- wash your hands after going to the toilet and before preparing food
- thaw out food slowly and thoroughly
- keep food either very cool or very hot
- keep cooked food separate from uncooked food
- keep everything in the kitchen very clean
- don't lick your fingers when handling food
- don't cough or sneeze over food.

What should you do about cleanliness?

People who handle food either in shops, food factories, kitchens or restaurants need to be especially responsible about the way they handle food. In shops where fresh food is sold, shop assistants must not handle food directly. Tongs are used for handling food. Furthermore, shop assistants must not handle both food and money, as the money may carry bacteria.

Some people can carry disease-producing organisms around with them and not realize it because they are not affected by them. These people are called **carriers** and they can cause an **epidemic** of a particular disease. If they cannot be cured of their disease they are not allowed to work where food is prepared or served.

One of the easiest ways to reduce the spread of diseases by food is for people to wash their hands before handling food. At school, at home and at work there should always be adequate washing facilities. All employers have a legal responsibility to provide employees with adequate toilet and washing facilities. This is particularly important if you work where food is manufactured or served.

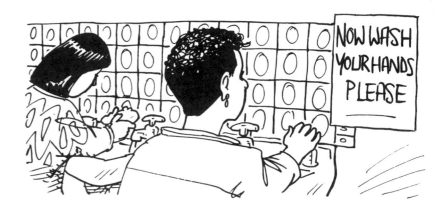

1 What is meant by the 'sell-by' date?
2 Why should you wash fruit before eating it?
3 How can you kill microbes which might be in a meat pie?
4 Why is it important to kill microbes in food?
5 What are the symptoms of food poisoning?
6 List three ways of reducing the risk of food poisoning.
7 Why should you wash your hands before handling food?
8 What is a 'carrier'?

Unit 7

Contamination of Food

Which animals contaminate food?

Food can become contaminated if it is affected by harmful microbes, such as bacteria and fungi during any stage of preparation, storage or distribution. The major carriers of these microbes are insects and rats.

Houseflies

Houseflies can contaminate food in various ways. They spray food with saliva, drop faeces and transfer microbes from decaying faeces onto food, and vomit partly digested food back onto the food. Houseflies also breed on rotting food. You should always keep food covered to stop flies landing on the food and transferring diseases such as dysentery, typhoid and cholera.

To control houseflies it is important that you:

- keep all food covered
- put the lid on dustbins
- destroy houseflies in the kitchen by swatting or using a fly spray
- keep all work tops and surfaces clean so there is no food exposed for houseflies
- clean the toilet regularly with disinfectant to prevent smells attracting flies.

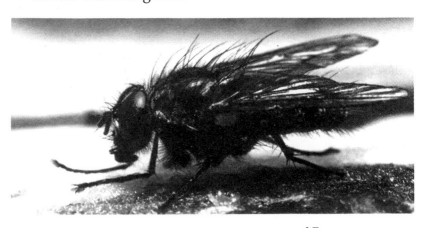

Keep all food covered to stop flies spreading disease.

Cockroaches

Cockroaches are another type of insect which may infect food. They carry bacteria to food and in doing so they transmit disease. Cockroaches live in warm kitchens, especially behind pipes and cookers, in cupboards and drawers.

They can be got rid of by:

- making sure that there are no food scraps left for cockroaches to feed on
- using insecticides which kill cockroaches.

Watch out for cockroaches in the kitchen.

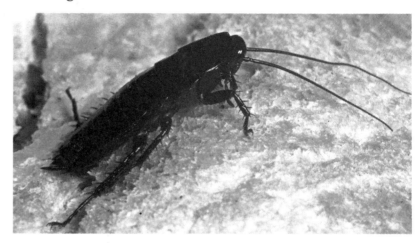

Ants

Ants often come indoors during hot weather and they too can carry bacteria which will contaminate food. There are various types of ant killers but you need to be very careful about how you use them, especially if you have young children or pets. You should carefully follow the instructions which are printed on the container. Ants can be got rid of by following the same basic advice as was given above for cockroaches.

Rats

Rats can be a dangerous source of contamination. They eat food, leave droppings on food and spread bacteria and fungi. In addition, rats carry fleas which themselves carry these disease-causing organisms. The dangers from rats can be reduced by:

- covering all food
- storing rubbish in strong dustbins with tight lids
- sealing up openings and cracks through which rats can enter buildings
- using rat traps or rat poison.

Contact the Pest Control Officer if you see a rat near your home.

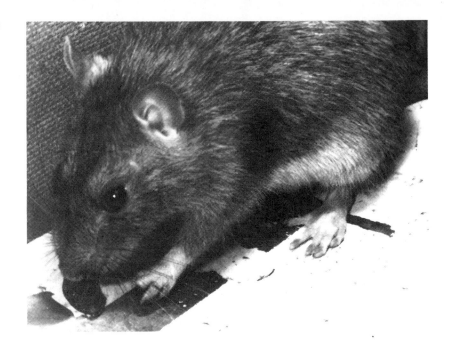

The local council will have a Pest Control Officer who will help you get rid of rats if you approach the council for advice.

1 Why should you always cover food?
2 How can the spread of houseflies be controlled?
3 Why are cockroaches harmful to Man?
4 What should you do if you have rats in your home?
5 How can you control insect pests such as ants or cockroaches?

Unit 8 | Infectious Diseases

What are infectious diseases?

If you get a disease from someone else then you have caught an infectious disease. Influenza ('flu) is one of the commonest infectious diseases.

Most diseases are caused by bacteria, viruses, fungi or very small one-celled organisms called protozoa and these can enter your body through your skin, mouth, nose or reproductive organs.

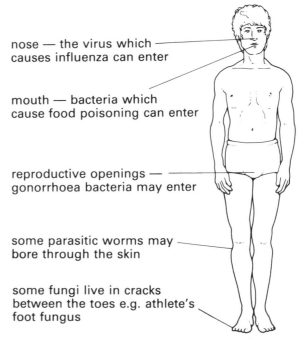

nose — the virus which causes influenza can enter

mouth — bacteria which cause food poisoning can enter

reproductive openings — gonorrhoea bacteria may enter

some parasitic worms may bore through the skin

some fungi live in cracks between the toes e.g. athlete's foot fungus

There are many ways in whch disease-causing organisms can enter your body.

When one of these organisms enters your body it begins to grow and reproduce very quickly. Your body immediately reacts to it and this reaction often causes the signs and symptoms of the disease. The sign of the disease can be seen by a doctor, for example, a rash is a sign of measles; the symptoms of a disease cannot be seen, they can only be described by the person who has the disease. Common symptoms of disease include high temperature, headache and pain.

How can you protect yourself against disease?

One way of preventing disease is to become **immune** to the disease. When you are immune it means that your blood contains antibodies which are special chemical substances produced by your own body to destroy the organisms that cause the disease.

Protection for babies and children

Babies have a **natural immunity** to some infectious diseases which they get from their mother while developing inside her. When a baby is born its blood already contains antibodies and more develop quite quickly, especially if the baby is breast fed because breast milk contains even more antibodies. As you grow older, your immunity gradually increases as your body produces more antibodies in response to the presence of bacteria and viruses in your body. When bacteria or viruses enter your body for the first time you may get the disease caused by them. However, while the disease is in your body, you will make antibodies which will make you immune and prevent you having the disease again.

After immunization you develop antibodies to protect you against disease.

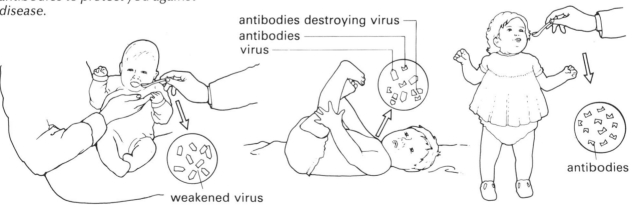

antibodies destroying virus
antibodies
virus

weakened virus

antibodies

The weakened virus is given to a young baby

Antibodies are produced in the baby's blood: the virus is destroyed.

More antibodies are produced when another dose of virus is given.

Immunization

When you were younger you probably had vaccinations from a doctor. The vaccine injected contained a very small amount of a weakened form of the bacteria or viruses which cause a particular disease, and this enabled your body to become immune to the particular disease by producing antibodies. This process is called **immunization**.

Find out which diseases you have been immunized against. Most babies are immunized against diphtheria, tetanus, whooping cough and polio. At about the age of 13 years you were probably immunized against tuberculosis. Girls of 14 years old are usually immunized against German measles, as exposure to this disease when they are pregnant could cause harm to their babies.

Table showing which immunizations you should have had.

Age	Immunization
From 3 months	Diptheria Whooping cough Tetanus Polio
5–6 months	Diphtheria Whooping cough Tetanus Polio
9–11 months	Diphtheria Whooping cough Tetanus Polio
12–24 months	Measles
About 5 years	Diphtheria (booster) Tetanus (booster) Polio (booster)
Girls of ages 10–14	Rubella (German measles)
Girls and boys at about 13 years	Tuberculosis
15–19 years (Leaving school)	Tetanus Polio

Different antibodies produce immunity which lasts for different lengths of time. For example, antibodies against polio last throughout life whereas those against tetanus are effective for five to ten years. After this time you need a 'booster' injection which will make your body produce more antibodies and give you inbuilt protection for a further ten years.

If, however, you are unfortunate enough to get a disease such as tetanus, you can receive an injection of **serum** which contains ready-made antibodies. These antibodies destroy the disease-causing organism and help you to recover quickly from the disease. This type of immunization is really only for emergencies and does not give any long-term protection. For example, if you cut yourself deeply on a rusty nail, tetanus bacteria may enter your body and cause death. An injection of ready-made antibodies destroys the tetanus bacteria and protects you for a few weeks afterwards.

If you go abroad on holiday you may be advised to be immunized against typhoid, cholera and yellow fever.

It may be unpleasant or inconvenient to have injections, but it is much worse if you actually get a disease. 5000 children died of diphtheria in England in 1911. Today this figure has been reduced to zero, thanks to a very successful programme of immunization.

Some parents today are refusing to have their children vaccinated against whooping cough as there is an extremely slight risk that the vaccine may cause brain damage in certain children. Consequently, there are now lots of children who are not protected against whooping cough and an epidemic could break out easily. Once a child has the disease it is too late to immunize against it. In 1982 there were 50 000 cases of whooping cough and 30 children died.

There are some risks therefore in being vaccinated and some risks in not being vaccinated. It is a decision which parents have to take.

How are diseases spread?

When there are large numbers of children who have not been immunized against a disease it can spread quickly through a population. This rapid spreading of a disease is called an **epidemic** and these were quite common right up to the middle of this century. Fortunately, as a result of immunization on a large scale, many worldwide diseases are now under control. For example, smallpox, which caused the plagues in the Middle Ages, has now been completely destroyed. No more smallpox viruses exist.

1 Why is 'flu described as an infectious illness?
2 List the four different types of disease-producing organism.
3 How can these organisms enter your body?
4 Describe two common symptoms of a disease.
5 What are antibodies?
6 Why are babies immune to disease a few weeks after birth?
7 When you have been immunized why do you sometimes need a booster injection?
8 What is likely to happen if a large number of children are not immunized against whooping cough?

Sexually transmitted diseases (STD's)

People who have sexual intercourse with several different partners, especially people who they don't know, are likely to get a sexually transmitted disease (STD). These are sometimes referred to as **venereal diseases** (VD). Every week over 3000 new cases of sexually transmitted disease are reported. These diseases can be very painful and make you feel uncomfortable. They can sometimes make you unable to have children later in life.

If you suspect that you have a sexually transmitted disease after having intercourse with someone who could have a disease you will need to go to a special clinic at your local hospital. You will find the address and telephone number in the yellow pages of the phone book under 'Clinics, STD'. Sometimes there is an STD answering service. You do not need a letter from your doctor before you go. The people at the clinic are very concerned to help you and will do all they can to treat you sympathetically.

You will need to tell the doctor for how long you have had the symptoms and what type of sexual contact you have had. You may need to give a urine or blood sample, and you may need to have your genital area examined. All information is treated in confidence.

So how are you supposed to know if you have a sexually transmitted disease?

- Have you had a sexual relationship with more than one partner?
- Have you had a sexual relationship with someone who may have had sex with several other people?
- Do you have any itching, soreness or discharge from the vagina or penis?
- Do you have any sores, lumps or rashes in the genital area?
- Do you need to pass urine often and feel uncomfortable at the time?

If you have any of these symptoms stop all sexual activity immediately and get medical advice.

More people have sexually transmitted diseases now than at any time in the last twenty years. STD's affect all ages and all social classes. One in every 400 people aged 15–19 has a sexually transmitted disease. Two of the commonest STD's are gonorrhoea and syphilis.

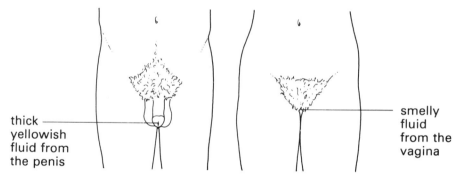

thick yellowish fluid from the penis

smelly fluid from the vagina

Visit the doctor if you have an unusual discharge from your penis or vagina.

So how are they spread?

The bacteria that cause gonorrhoea and syphilis are spread during direct sexual contact of any kind, such as:

- sexual intercourse (penis – vagina)
- anal contact (penis – anus)
- oral contact (genital – mouth).

Every week 1000 people in Britain catch **gonorrhoea**. It is the second most common disease after measles. You cannot become immune to gonorrhoea but it can be cured. It is up to you whether or not you are re-infected.

Male	Female
Pain when passing water, yellow discharge from penis.	Unusual vaginal discharge, burning feeling when passing water, fever symptoms, painful joints.

If you do not get treatment then more serious complications occur. In men the testes become infected, the sperm tubes are blocked and the man is unable to father a child.

In women the womb and egg tubes become inflamed and then blocked and the woman is unable to have children.

There may be permanent damage to the reproductive organs and to the blood stream in men and women.

Syphilis is one of the most serious sexually transmitted diseases. If it is not diagnosed it can develop into a chronic crippling disease leading to death.

You may find symptoms appearing ten days to twelve weeks after infection. The symptoms are the same in men and women and occur in four stages:

1. A painless sore on the sex organ, or even inside the rectum or vagina.
2. Body rash, mouth sores, flu-like symptoms and a feeling of ill health.
3. No symptoms but the disease can be detected by blood tests.
4. Serious damage to heart, eyes, ears, nervous system leading to death.

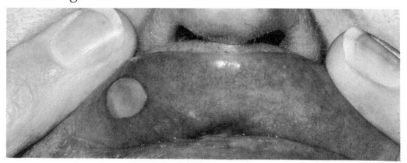

One of the first signs of syphilis may be a painless sore inside the mouth.

It is possible for treatment of syphilis to be effective at most stages of the disease but it is very important not to have sexual contact with anyone until the disease is no longer infectious. The most usual treatment is a course of antibiotics, for example, penicillin.

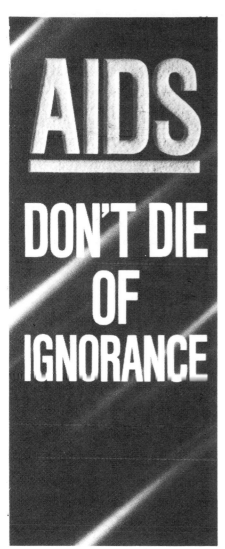

AIDS

The most serious disease to be spread by unprotected sexual intercourse is AIDS (Acquired Immune Deficiency Syndrome). AIDS is thought to be caused by a virus called HIV which stands for Human Immune Deficiency Virus. HIV reduces the body's ability to fight infection and disease and may result in AIDS. The World Health Organisation (WHO) estimate that 8–10 million people are infected with the HIV virus in 1992. However, not all people with HIV develop AIDS. The reasons for this are not fully understood.

How can you become infected with HIV?

The HIV virus lives in body fluids such as blood, semen, saliva and tears. All known cases of HIV have been passed on through infected blood or semen. The virus can enter the body via the bloodstream, for example during unprotected sexual intercourse with an infected person, and there's no way of knowing who is infected. The more people you have intercourse with the greater the risk of contracting HIV. The virus can also be passed on from a mother to her baby through the placenta or breast milk.

Another way of getting the HIV virus is when drug users inject themselves with unsterilized needles (see Unit 4). Some people have caught the virus by having blood transfusions using blood from infected people. All blood is now tested and treated before being used for transfusions so there is less risk of this happening.

If you want more information about AIDS there are several leaflets which you can obtain from your local Health Centre. If you are worried about being infected you should visit your doctor or local STD Clinic.

Other diseases spread by sexual contact

Trichomoniasis and non-specific urethritis (NSU) are two other diseases spread by sexual contact. They cause an abnormal discharge from the penis and vagina and soreness on passing urine. These diseases can be cured by taking a course of tablets prescribed by the doctor.

It is important to realize that if you have a stable relationship with your partner you are most unlikely to get a sexually transmitted disease. If you have casual sex with different partners who you do not know there is a very good chance that you will develop a sexually transmitted disease. Sexually transmitted diseases are therefore diseases linked with promiscuous sexual behaviour and can affect people at any time in their life, not just young people.

---

1 When should you visit a special clinic at the hospital?
2 What are the outward signs of a sexually transmitted disease?
3 What are the symptoms of gonorrhoea in a male and a female?
4 Why is it important to get treatment for sexually transmitted diseases?
5 Why are you more likely to get a sexually transmitted disease if you are promiscuous than if you have a stable relationship with one person?

Parasites and animals which carry disease (vectors)

Parasites are small animals which feed on other animals which are called **hosts**. They live inside, or on the surface of, their host. Most parasites do not affect your health but there are some which cause serious diseases such as malaria, sleeping sickness, cholera and typhoid. In the Middle Ages a parasite caused one third of the population of Europe to die of bubonic plague. The parasites which caused the plague were bacteria which were passed from rats to humans by fleas. These bacteria caused disease in both rats and humans but not in fleas which acted only as the means of *transmitting* the disease from one animal to another animal. Organisms which do this are called **vectors**.

There are a number of common parasites which affect humans and they are transferred directly from person to person without help from a vector. These parasites include the ones described below.

It is wise to keep children's finger nails short so that if they scratch their bottoms they are less likely to pick up threadworm eggs.

How do vectors transmit disease?

Some parasites are carried by animals. For example, the mosquito carries tiny single-celled parasitic organisms which cause malaria. The mosquito transfers the parasites into the person's blood and the parasites enter the liver and then the blood stream. The effect on the person is to have a very severe fever, which can result in death.

Mosquitoes also transfer viruses which cause yellow fever and dengue fever.

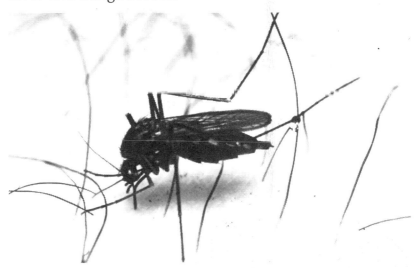

The female mosquito carries the parasite which causes malaria.

Control of parasites

There are two main methods of controlling parasites.

Firstly you can stop the parasite reaching its host, and secondly you can treat the parasite when it has reached its host.

1. Preventing infection

Many countries require you to have been immunized against a particular disease before entering the country so that you do not bring the disease-causing parasites into the country.

When animals are brought into this country they are kept in special areas for a particular length of time. During this time they are watched closely to ensure that they do not develop diseases. This treatment is called **quarantine**. Once the animals are certified as being free from disease they can leave their temporary quarters and rejoin their owners.

The Public Health Authority checks the import and export of meat to make sure that it is free of parasites. If contaminated meat came into the country it could cause an outbreak of a disease such as foot and mouth disease and thousands of farm animals would have to be destroyed. When animals are slaughtered the meat is usually checked to see if it contains parasites.

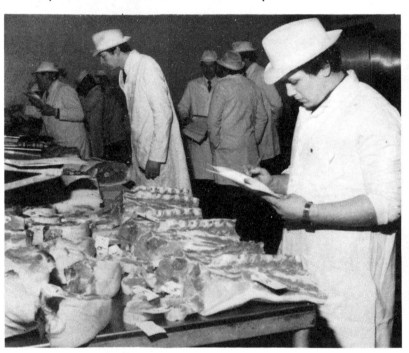

An inspector checks that the meat you will eat does not contain parasites.

Good hygiene and safe disposal of faeces also helps to control the spread of parasites. When meat is thoroughly cooked the parasites are destroyed, and when milk is pasteurized all the harmful bacteria are destroyed.

2. Treating infection

When animals become infected with a parasite they can be treated with chemicals to help destroy the parasite. For example, sheep and cattle are completely immersed in a dip tank which contains a solution which destroys many mites, ticks and fleas.

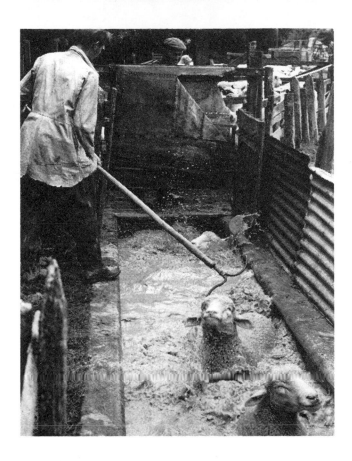

The liquid in the tank destroys the parasites.

There are many drugs available to help treat humans who have parasites but these drugs often have unpleasant side-effects. Sometimes the parasites become resistant to the drug and a new treatment has to be developed as has occurred several times in the case of the malarial parasite.

1 Name two diseases caused by parasites.
2 How could you find out if you have head lice?
3 What should you do if you have head lice?
4 What causes scabies?
5 How can you stop children getting 'worms'?
6 What causes malaria and what transmits the disease?
7 Why does the Public Health Authority inspect meat?
8 How can a farmer prevent sheep getting parasites?

Unit 9

Environmental Hazards

You should be aware of the health problems which can result from harmful disturbances and substances in your surroundings. There are many forms of **pollution** in the environment but there are four main forms which may have a direct bearing on your health. These are noise, dust, fibres and radiation.

Noise

'You are making too much noise', or 'I can't stand that noise any longer'. These two everyday comments may help you understand what we mean by the word noise. Sounds which become too loud or annoy people can be described as noise. All noise or sound is really vibrations of the air which hit the ear drum and cause the ear drum to vibrate. These vibrations are transmitted to the brain and you interpret the sounds. Sometimes we need to be able to describe the loudness of a sound. Sound is measured in units called **decibels** using a sound meter or decibel meter. One decibel (db) is about the smallest amount of sound that you can detect. Very loud noise can be extremely unpleasant and harmful to your ears.

Sometimes people have to work in very noisy factories or other places where there is noisy machinery. It is possible to suffer hearing damage which may lead to deafness if you are subjected to excessive noise at work. The recommended upper level for noise at work is 85 decibels. About this level your employer should provide you with ear defenders to protect your ears, and you should make sure that you actually wear them if you work in a noisy place.

Pop music can also cause damage to your ears. If you stand near an amplifier at a disco you will usually find that you cannot hear well for several hours or days afterwards. You are not usually aware of the damage that is being caused to your ears at the time.

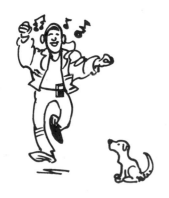

Several hours of this could damage your hearing.

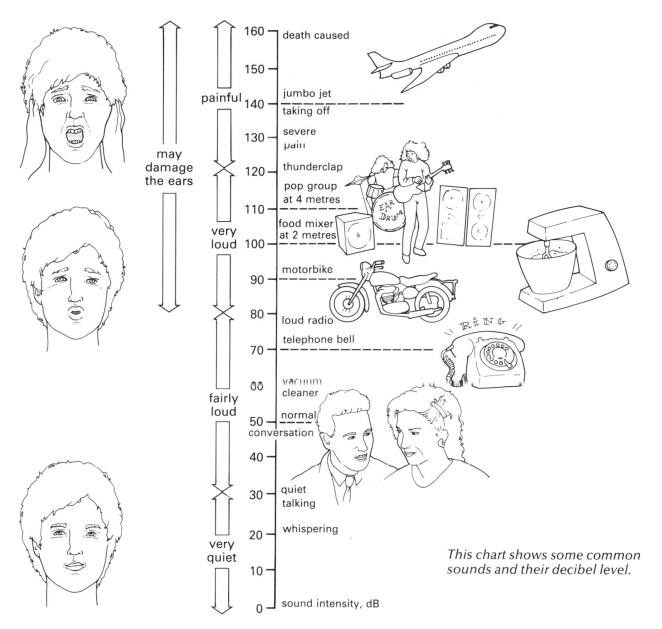

painful	160	death caused
	150	
	140	jumbo jet taking off
	130	severe pain
	120	thunderclap
	110	pop group at 4 metres
very loud	100	food mixer at 2 metres
	90	motorbike
	80	loud radio
	70	telephone bell
fairly loud	60	vacuum cleaner
	50	normal conversation
	40	
	30	quiet talking
	20	whispering
very quiet	10	
	0	sound intensity, dB

may damage the ears

This chart shows some common sounds and their decibel level.

If you are subjected to noise over 97 decibels for more than three hours a day you will suffer from temporary deafness or even permanent deafness. Listening to a personal stereo for several hours a day can also affect your eardrums. You may find that after a while you will not be able to hear sounds at high frequencies. The stress resulting from noise over about 90 decibels can cause your arteries to constrict and put a strain on your heart. Investigations have also shown that people who live near airports are eight times more likely to suffer from mental stress than people who live in quieter areas.

So how can you protect yourself against noise?

- Wear ear defenders if you work in or near a noisy environment.
- Don't stand near amplifiers at a disco.
- Reduce the volume and listening time with your personal headphones.
- Try to obtain a grant for double glazing if you live near a noisy road or airport.
- Identify the source of irritating or loud noise and see if anything can be done to reduce the noise at its source.

---

1 What are 'noises' or sounds?
2 Draw a flow chart to show how sounds are detected by the ear and sent to the brain.
3 What instrument would you use to measure how loud a sound is?
4 What is the recommended maximum level for noise at work?
5 What are two causes of temporary deafness?
6 List three ways of protecting yourself against excessive noise.

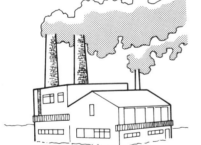

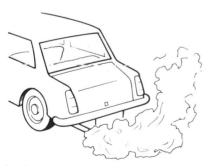

The air you breathe in contains waste gases from chimneys and car exhausts.

Air pollution—dust and fibres

Every time you breathe in you take in air which has many things in it apart from the gases normally found in the atmosphere, (nitrogen, oxygen and carbon dioxide). The air will contain waste gases from burning fuels, such as sulphur dioxide, carbon monoxide and nitrogen dioxide, as well as particles of dust and soot, smoke, and even lead. These are all pollutants.

What is the effect of air pollutants on your health?

If you live near a factory such as a cement works, you will often see large white clouds of dust in the air which you, in turn, breathe in. However, everyone breathes in dust which has been blown about in the wind but most of this is harmless and is collected up in the mucus in your air tubes and lungs, passed into your throat and swallowed. If you breathe in a lot of dust, or dust which is toxic, your lungs produce too much mucus which you can only remove by coughing. This can lead to **bronchitis**. People who smoke or who have asthma also have difficulty in breathing and if they live or work in a dusty environment are more likely to get bronchitis. About 30 000 people die of bronchitis every year in the United Kingdom.

We all breathe in many very small particles but they are usually filtered out by the hairs and mucus of the air tubes and lungs. Some particles however reach the tiny airsacs (alveoli) deep inside the lungs and can cause damage. The two types of particles which can cause serious damage are silica and asbestos.

If your job involves cutting, grinding or drilling rock you may be exposed to **silica dust**. The silica particles collect in your lungs and become surrounded by scar tissues made up of dead cells. Your lungs then become stiff and you find it harder to breathe. Eventually you may develop the disease **silicosis**.

You should make sure that you wear the correct breathing apparatus, such as a mask or face shield. Many jobs involving silica should be carried out in the presence of water which reduces the amount of dust in the air.

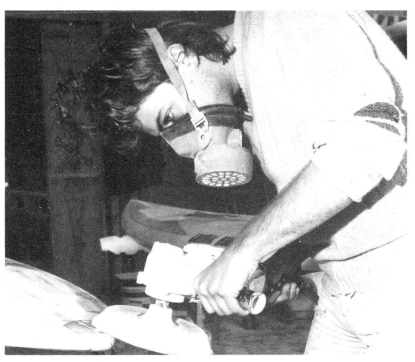

The correct apparatus should be worn to protect the lungs from dust.

If you breathe in **asbestos dust** it will harm your lungs. The dust is made up of tiny fibres which can cause **abestosis** and **lung cancer**. Asbestos used to be thought of as a harmless substance and people used no protective breathing equipment when they handled asbestos. People who smoke cigarettes and work with asbestos are very likely to suffer from lung cancer.

You need only have breathed in asbestos fibres for a few months to increase the risk of having lung cancer.

The main problem in handling asbestos arises when old asbestos has to be removed from buildings where it has been used to insulate walls and ceilings. It is essential that if you are going to be working with asbestos you are fully protected against breathing in the fibres.

1 List three pollutants which are in the air that you breathe in.
2 How does your body get rid of dust particles which you breathe in?
3 Which pollutant can cause bronchitis?
4 What is the effect of silica particles in your lungs?
5 What precautions should you use if your job involves working with asbestos?

Radiation

Your health can be affected by radiation and you need to understand the risks involved. For example, if you work in a hospital or as a dental nurse you may be involved in taking X-rays of patients. It is essential that you protect yourself by standing behind a metal screen or by wearing a lead apron. The X-rays affect the ovaries and testes. Exposure to X-rays over a period of time can affect the development of the egg cells and sperm cells and lead to sterility. Women who are pregnant should avoid having X-rays as they can affect the growing fetus.

Nuclear power stations have very high safety levels and everyone who works in a nuclear power station is monitored to check the amount of radiation which they are exposed to every year. The main risk from radiation to ordinary people comes from the disposal of nuclear waste. High-level radioactive waste is usually dumped at sea in lead and concrete containers. Medium- and low-level radioactive waste is usually buried underground.

However, there is growing concern being expressed about the risk of these radioactive wastes contaminating water and land.

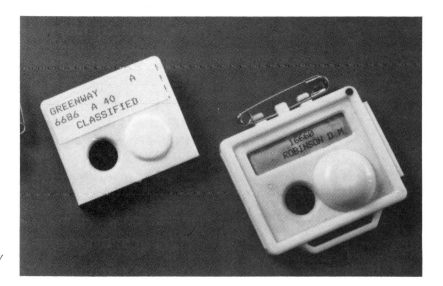

These badges are checked regularly to monitor the radiation level.

---

1 What precaution should you take if your job involves you using an X-ray machine?
2 What is the effect of X-rays on the ovaries and testes?
3 Why are radiation levels checked at a power station?
4 What happens to radioactive waste?

SAFETY
Unit 10 Safety at Work

Accidents can occur anywhere and any time in your everyday life. You should be aware of the potential hazards, and the safety precautions which you should take, at work, at home and when using the roads.

The law

About 250 000 people are injured and over 600 people die every year from accidents at work. Your place of work may be an office, shop, garage, factory, or building site but wherever you work safety is very important.

There are several Acts of Parliament which are involved with safety at work, the most important Act being the **Health and Safety at Work Act** passed in 1974. This Act contains information about the responsibilities and duties of employers and employees so that everyone can be involved in reducing the number of accidents at work.

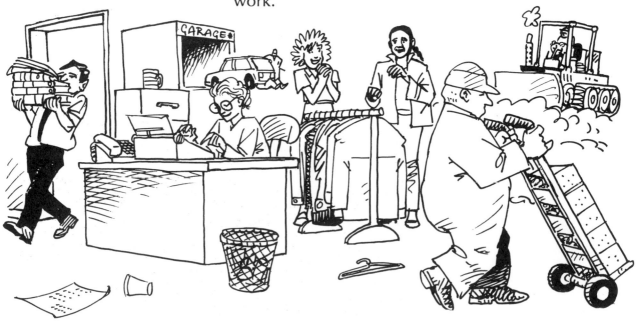

Duties of employers

It is the duty of every employer to ensure, as far as possible, the health, safety and welfare at work of their employees. This means that your employer has a responsibility to you to take reasonable care of your safety. If you are injured while employed by someone you may be able to sue your employer in court for compensation for your injuries.

Here is a summary list of some of an employer's main responsibilities. The employer should:

- keep the rooms clean
- prevent overcrowding — each person must have about 3.5 m³ space
- keep a reasonable temperature, usually above 16°C
- ensure good ventilation and lighting
- provide suitable toilet facilities
- keep the toilets clean and properly maintained
- provide suitable washing facilities with soap, hot and cold water and a method of drying hands
- provide a supply of drinking water, and facilities for eating meals.

The purpose of all these regulations is to make sure that employees have good conditions for working in.

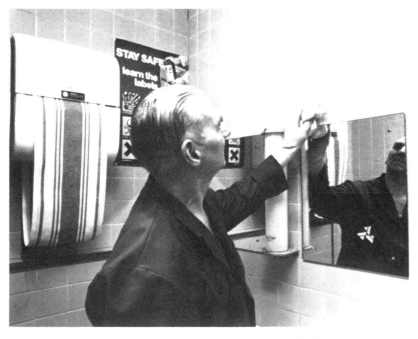

An employer must provide washing facilities and keep them clean and properly maintained.

Employers also need to be aware of safety and the possible hazards which exist in your place of work. Your employer must:

- check that you are trained and competent to do the work
- check that you are not a risk to other employees
- provide the correct equipment for the job
- check that you take reasonable care of the equipment
- provide you with a safe place to work
- provide you with the correct protective clothing and protective materials
- fence in all dangerous machinery
- provide first aid kits and someone trained in first aid
- provide fire-fighting equipment and ensure that all employees know what to do in the event of a fire (see Unit 11).

Duties of employees

When you are employed by an employer you must take reasonable care for your own safety. If you disregard the safety rules and contribute to an injury to yourself then you may get only a reduced amount of damages awarded to you by the court.

When you work for someone else you have certain responsibilities. Here is a summary list. You should:

- take reasonable care of your own health and safety
- take reasonable care of the health and safety of people who may be working with you
- cooperate with your employer in matters of health and safety
- not interfere with equipment which has been provided for health and safety.

---

1 What Act was passed in 1974 to help prevent accidents at work?
2 List three responsibilities of an employer.
3 List three responsibilities of an employee.

Fire Precautions

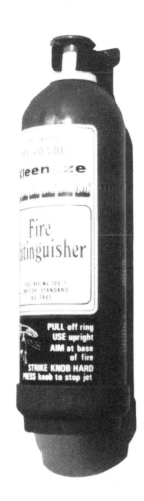

Any place where several people meet together, for example, a school, cinema, factory or office, must have adequate fire precautions. These places require a Fire Certificate which is issued after the building has been inspected by the Fire Brigade when they are satisfied that the fire precautions have reached the required standard.

Fire precautions at work

In your place of work it is the responsibility of your employer to provide the necessary fire-fighting equipment and to ensure that you, as an employee, know what to do in the event of a fire.

In particular your place of work should have:

● adequate fire escapes which are clearly labelled
● a sufficient number of conveniently placed fire alarms
● adequate fire-fighting equipment, for example, fire buckets filled with sand, fire blankets, fire extinguishers
● one person responsible for all matters related to safety in the event of a fire
● adequate fire drills.

Fire precautions in the home

In your home you should know the basic safety rules which apply to heating appliances such as cookers, electric fires, oil and gas heaters, and electric blankets.

If you ignore the safety precautions then a serious fire could occur in your home which could injure or kill you, your family or your pets.

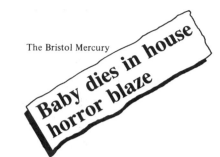

Pensioners die in home fire

The Bristol Mercury

Baby dies in house horror blaze

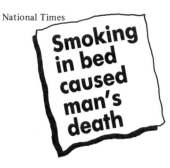

Smoking in bed caused man's death

Family of five in fire

How do you prevent fires starting at home?

It is difficult to stop fires once they have started. It is much easier to prevent a fire starting. Here are some ways you can take responsibility for fire prevention at home:

- keep matches away from children
- don't leave children on their own especially where there is an open fire, a heating appliance or cooker
- never leave a chip pan unattended and remember to only half fill the pan with oil or fat
- keep curtains and clothes away from cookers and heaters as they can easily catch light
- make sure all fires have a guard over them
- check the house at night – switch off TV sets, heaters, record players and pull out the plugs, check ashtrays for burning cigarettes
- close all doors.

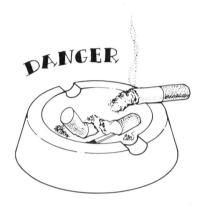

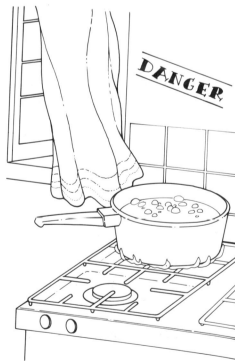

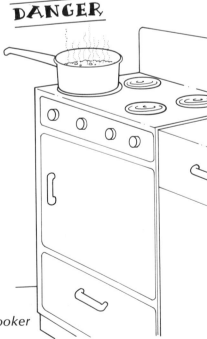

Never leave the handles of saucepans hanging over the cooker where they may be knocked.

But if fire does break out....

■ Make sure the door of the room where the fire is located is closed— this will help to contain the fire and restrict the spread of poisonous fumes.

■ Warn the household and get everyone out by the safest route.

■ Call the fire brigade by dialling 999 (don't leave it to somebody else). You don't need to put money in a public phone box. Remember to give the full address of the fire.

■ Don't go back in for any reason.

Advice given by the Central Office of Information.

In an emergency situation, such as a fire or an accident, you need to remain calm and think very clearly. People often panic when involved in an emergency, and are unable to think sensibly. Just by being clear-headed you could save someone's life.

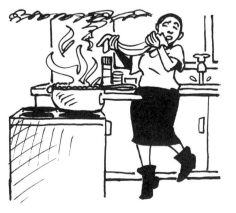

Chip pan fires

In case of a chip pan fire

- put a damp cloth or lid over the pan of oil
- turn off the heat
- leave the pan to cool before trying to move it
- don't try to carry a blazing chip pan out of the house because the air will help the flames to burn, and you may trip over
- don't pour water onto the oil as this will spread the oil and spread the flames.

Clothing

Follow these guidelines:

- if someone's clothes are on fire get them to lie down and cover them with a thick blanket or rug, in order to stop air from getting to the flames
- if you cannot find anything to cover them with, roll the person over to put out the flames.

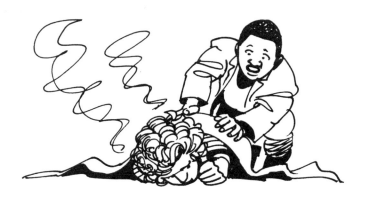

Some basic safety rules when using cooking and heating appliances

There are many places in the home where fires can start. The majority of fires begin because people ignore basic rules concerning the use of cookers, heaters and open fires. Here are some of the basic safety precautions which should be taken when using cooking and heating appliances.

Electric cookers

An electric cooker cannot be plugged into an ordinary 13 amp socket because it uses a high current of electricity supplied by a very thick electric cable. An electric cooker therefore needs its own power supply and should be connected to the electrical supply by a qualified electrician.

Gas cookers

Gas cookers need to be connected by a Gas Board fitter to make sure that the gas supply is safe and that there is adequate ventilation. (See also under Gas fires for special safety rules relating to the use of gas.)

Electric fires

Make sure that:

- the fire has a guard over the element so that children cannot easily burn themselves
- the fire is connected to the electric socket using a 3-pin plug to earth the appliance
- the flex joining the fire and socket is placed behind the fire where it cannot be tripped over
- all clothes, bedding and furniture are kept away from the fire.

Remember to keep the rule:

one appliance, one socket

How many hazards can you see in this room?

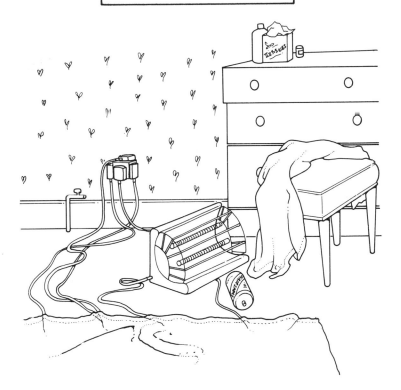

Gas fires

There are many different types of gas fire. Some are fixed to the main gas supply, others are portable gas heaters which use bottled gas which is stored under pressure in heavy gas cylinders.

As with any fire you should make sure that:

- there is a guard over the front of the heater to prevent clothes and curtains from coming into contact with the flames

- you are ready to light the heater when you switch it on by checking that the pilot light is alight, or by having a match ready if your heater does not have a pilot light
- if your gas heater works from a slot meter you have turned off the gas before you put money in the meter.

If you smell gas you should know what action to take as follows:

- turn out all flames and put out cigarettes
- open the windows and doors to let in fresh air
- check to see if a gas tap has been left on
- if you think there is a gas leak turn off the main gas tap and contact the Gas service — the telephone number is in the phone book under Gas.

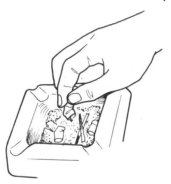

If you think there is a gas leak stub out cigarettes immediately and turn the main gas tap off.

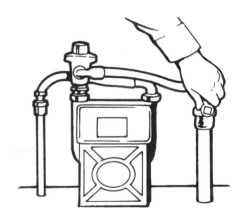

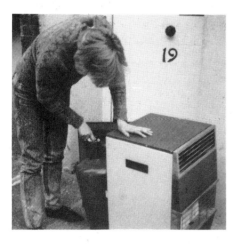

Change the gas cylinder outside.

Portable gas heaters

There are special precautions you should take when using any portable gas heater. One of the most important to remember is never to move the heater when it is alight. When you have to change the gas cylinder you should take the heater outside, or at least open all the windows and doors to ensure a good air supply. You should change the cylinder only when the old cylinder is empty and the heater is switched off. You should store any spare gas cylinders outside if possible, but if you have to keep them indoors store them away from sources of heat.

Paraffin heaters

Some people who live in rural areas use paraffin heaters. These are potentially very dangerous because paraffin is a liquid fuel which can catch light very easily. Therefore you should:

- keep paraffin in correctly labelled metal containers which have a screw top
- keep the containers of paraffin in a locked shed or garage
- always take the heater outside to fill it and check you are using the correct fuel
- don't leave the heater in a draught or where it causes an obstruction and could be knocked over.

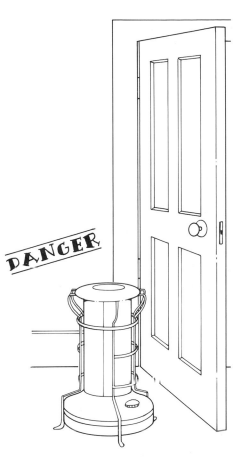

Open fires

You should take these precautions with open fires:

- all fires should have a large guard over them, especially where there are children who are fascinated by flames
- don't put things on the shelf or mantelpiece over the fire in case they get knocked off and catch alight, for example, Christmas cards
- don't store fuel next to the fire because the fuel can ignite.

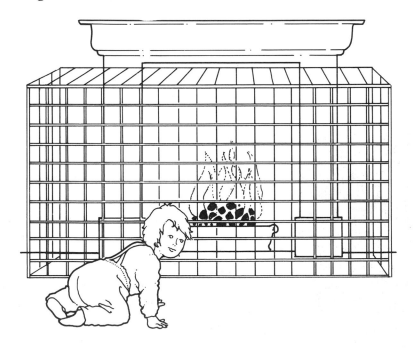

Electric blankets

Many people use electric blankets to heat their bed in winter. There are two types of blanket, underblankets which go underneath the bottom sheet, and over-blankets which go over you in bed.

There are a number of safety precautions which you should take when using an underblanket:

- always switch off your electric blanket before getting into bed
- always tie the blanket securely in place using the correct tapes and loops on the blanket
- don't tuck in the wired area of the blanket.

Follow these guidelines when using an overblanket:

- some of these may be left on when you are in bed
- only use a light cover over the electric blanket
- don't tuck in the wired area
- check the blanket is laid flat on the bed.

With either type of blanket use a 3 amp fuse (see Unit 12) in the 3-pin plug. If there is a fault in the blanket the fuse will break or 'blow' and stop the electricity flowing. There is less chance of a fire starting if there is no electricity reaching the blanket. Have all electric blankets checked by the manufacturer every two years.

You should not use an electric blanket if you are in the final stages of pregnancy or if you are incontinent. At the end of pregnancy the fluid surrounding the baby may be unexpectedly released and this will wet the bed. Likewise, people who are incontinent cannot control their bladder and may wet the bed. Water conducts electricity and any bedwetting may cause the person in bed to be electrocuted.

You should not use an electric blanket which is very old, frayed or damaged — it can overheat and cause a fire. If the electric blanket causes a fire there are a number of things that you should do:

- immediately switch off and unplug the electric blanket
- try to put out the fire by covering the bed with a heavy blanket or rug.

If you are unable to put out the fire you must get everyone out of the house and call the Fire Brigade.

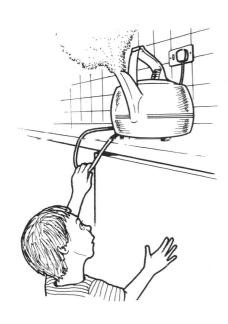

Prevention of burns and scalds

Children can burn and scald themselves very easily. For example, they may tip boiling water over themselves if they reach up to a cooker and grab the handle of a saucepan, or the flex of a kettle.

Children also like to play with matches and they do not understand how easily a fire can be started. If you have children in your care, perhaps when babysitting, it is your responsibility to prevent them causing injury to themselves.

Sometimes, however, accidents do happen and you should know some basic first aid so that you can give immediate treatment before getting the child to the doctor or hospital. You may decide that you want to learn more about first aid so that you know what to do in an emergency. Several organizations run courses for young people covering topics such as what to do in case of an accident, fire prevention and survival. Two of the most well-known organizations are the British Red Cross and the St John's Ambulance Brigade. Local Scout or Guide organizations also involve young people in learning about first aid.

Treatment of burns and scalds

1. Put the burn or scald immediately under cold water, or run plenty of cold water over the burn or scald. A young child can be placed in a washing up bowl of clean cold water. In this way the cold water takes the heat away from the skin. The burn or scald needs to be under cold water for at least ten minutes.
2. Remove any tight belts or rings. Burnt skin usually swells up.
3. Cover the skin very lightly with a non-fluffy cloth that is clean. A pillow case or clean linen tea towel could be used. This helps to cut down the danger of infection.
4. Don't try to take off burnt clothes which may be stuck to the skin.
5. Call an ambulance or take the child to hospital.
6. Don't put butter, oil or ointment on a burn. These can trap in the heat and cause more damage.

1 When you start work what information about fire precautions do you need to find out about?
2 What should you do if there is a fire at home?
3 List three ways of preventing a fire at home.
4 Look at the picture opposite — how many dangers you can spot?
5 Why does an electric cooker need a very thick cable?
6 What can happen to curtains which hang near a cooker?
7 How should you store paraffin?
8 What should you do if you smell gas?
9 What precaution must you take when using an electric fire?
10 When should you not use an electric blanket?
11 What should you do immediately someone has burned themselves?
12 Why is it a good idea to learn about first aid?
13 Name one organization which runs first aid courses. Find out how to contact them and when the next course is due to start.

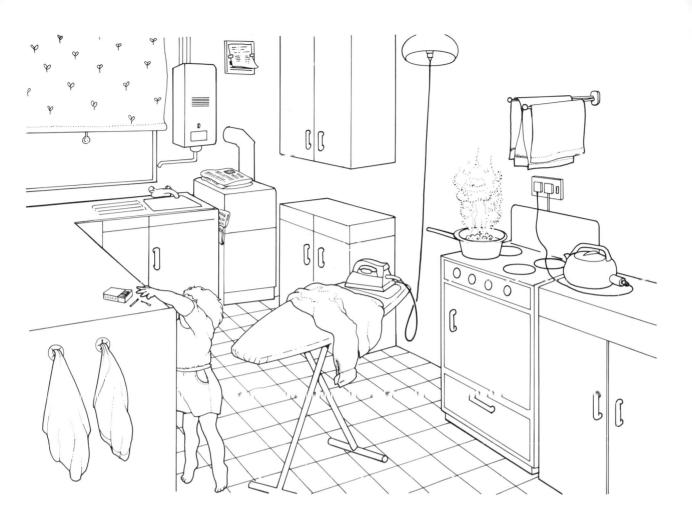

Spot the hazards in this kitchen.

Unit 12

Electricity in the Home

There are a number of safety precautions which you should take to reduce the risk of having an accident when using electricity. You should know how to fit a plug on to an electrical appliance, and what type of fuse to use. You should also know what to do if someone receives an electric shock as a result of an accident involving electricity.

Wiring a plug

When you buy an electrical appliance such as a record player, computer, kettle, electric drill or hair drier, it usually requires a plug on the end of the flex.

If you are going to connect a plug correctly to the flex you must be sure of what you are doing. The plug is usually supplied with a card reminding you of the correct colours but it's useful to learn the colour code used for wiring a plug correctly.

How to fix a plug to a cable
1. You will need a small screwdriver and a 3-pin plug with the correct fuse.
2. Usually the appliance has the ends of the wire stripped back so you can see the copper wire. If this has not been done you will need to cut the sleeve of the cable and trim away about 5 cm.
3. Push the flex under the cable grip and tighten the two cable grip screws.
4. Check the colour code shown below and cut the 3 wires to the right length.
5. Trim each wire so that the plastic insulation is removed. You should be able to see a short length of shiny copper wire. It can sometimes help to twist each copper wire so that the strands stay together.

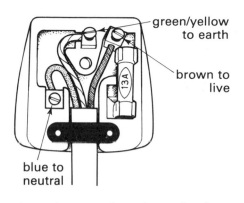

green/yellow
to earth

brown to
live

blue to
neutral

Learn how to wire a three-pin plug correctly.

6. Fix each wire to the correct pin and tighten each screw. You should not be able to see any bare wires.
7. Screw the back of the plug in place.

Remember: **the brown** wire fixes to the **live** pin
(on the right)
the **blue** wire fixes to the **neutral** pin
(on the left)
the **green** or **green/yellow** wire fixes to the **earth** pin (the one at the top)

Fuses

It is important to use the correct fuse in any electrical plug. This will ensure that the fuse will burn out or 'blow' before the appliance becomes dangerous. When an appliance is faulty, too much current can flow through it and cause damage. Using a fuse, therefore, protects you from danger. You should check that the plug contains the correct fuse for whichever electrical appliance you are going to use the plug. For example, a 3 amp fuse is required for a vacuum cleaner, a table lamp, and an electric blanket, whereas a 13 amp fuse is necessary for electric kettles, fires and television sets.

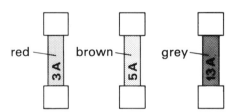

red   brown   grey

3 A   5 A   13 A

Fuses.

Some modern appliances are insulated so that any electricity that escapes will pass to the plastic around the appliance and will not reach you. These appliances are marked with a symbol:

Most appliances need to have an earth wire. The earth wire lets the current flow to earth and not to you if there is a fault in the appliance. The earth wire is a 'safety wire'.

Safety precautions

Take these precautions:

- always have dry hands when you touch an electrical appliance or switch
- always use a pull cord to switch on a light in a bathroom
- keep all electrical appliances out of the bathroom unless they are firmly fixed on a wall out of reach
- always use one electric appliance fixed to any one socket
- do not overload sockets — this can cause too much current to flow and the wires become overheated
- always switch off at the socket before removing a plug
- switch off electricity at the mains before doing any repair work
- never join together two pieces of flex without using a connector otherwise too much current will flow and the wires will overheat and cause a fire
- get a qualified electrician to do most of the repair work at home.

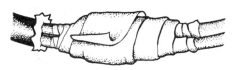

Overloading sockets is very dangerous.

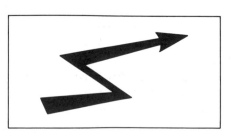

Always use a proper connector to join two pieces of flex together.

What is an electric shock?

If you follow all the safety precautions you should never have an electric shock. However, you may be present when someone suffers from an electric shock as a result of coming into contact with high or low voltages.

High-voltage injuries

These can be caused by coming into contact with over-head power cables, conductor rails of electric railways or in certain industries where high voltage is used.

If the person is still in contact with the high voltage do not attempt to touch the person. You must call the police and give them as much information as possible. Touch the person only when you are told that the supply is switched off and isolated from being accidentally switched on again. High voltages can spark across several metres distance so do not go near the person until it is safe.

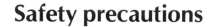

Warning sign for high voltage.

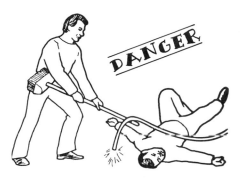

Keep well away from a person who has received an electric shock — the electricity could 'jump' across.

Low-voltage injuries

These are the result of coming into contact with the household electricity supply, e.g. someone who has cut through a lawnmower cable. You must switch off the electricity supply or break the contact between the person and the low voltage. You may be able to use a dry wooden broom handle or folded newspaper to push the person's limbs away from the electricity. Do not touch the person directly because you will receive a shock.

Treatment for someone suffering from an electric shock

When a person has suffered an electric shock, he or she may be injured and unconscious as a result of an electric current passing through the body. You should not touch the person until you are sure of the cause of the shock and you can make sure you will not get an electric shock. The person may have stopped breathing and the heart may have stopped beating. It is up to you to act quickly to help. You may be able to give **resuscitation** — artificial respiration (the 'kiss of life') and chest compression. If possible you should receive training in this method from the local Red Cross organization or St John's Ambulance Brigade.

It is best to call an ambulance or doctor when a person is in a state of shock.

Sometimes the person can suffer from burns where the electrical current entered and left the body. You will need to treat the burns if possible (see Unit 11).

---

1 When you wire a plug which colour wire fixes to the live pin?
2 Why is it important to fit the correct fuse into a plug?
3 What does this symbol mean? ☐
4 List three safety precautions you should use when using electricity.
5 What should you do if you find someone suffering from a high-voltage electric shock?
6 Describe briefly how you would give someone the kiss of life.

Safety in the Home

Many accidents occur in people's own homes. There are, however, certain groups of people who are at higher risk than others from accidents in the home, for example children, the elderly and the handicapped.

Prevention of accidents to children

There are many ways that a child can have an accident at home and if you are looking after a young child you should be aware of the potential hazards. Children have no idea that they can injure and harm themselves by playing with apparently harmless items.

The chart on the next page summarizes the main causes of accidents which usually involve children, how you could prevent an accident and what you should do if a child in your care is injured.

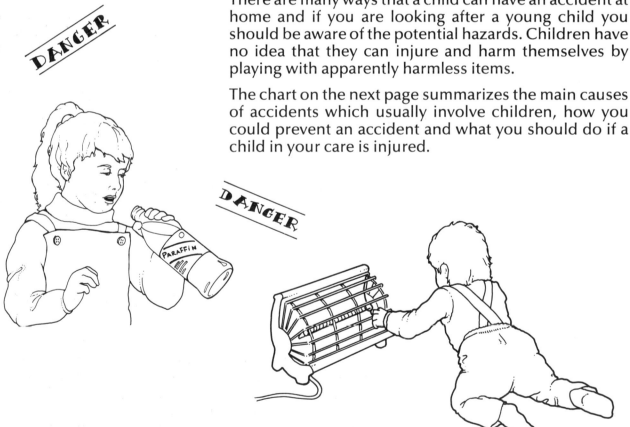

DANGER

DANGER

Problem	Cause	What to do	Prevention
Choking	Small objects in mouth.	Hold child upside down and slap their back.	Keep small objects out of reach of a child.
Suffocation	Plastic bag over head.	Take off bag, give mouth-to-mouth resuscitation, take child to hospital.	Keep polythene bags away from children.
Scalds	Tipping hot water over themselves.	Put burned area into cold water, take child to hospital.	Don't let handles stick out over the cooker.
Falls	Climbing bannisters or opening windows.	Don't move child, call ambulance, give mouth-to-mouth resuscitation if child has stopped breathing.	Use protective rails and window bars.
Poisoning	Child eats pills that look like sweets.	Call doctor or take to hospital, take pills with you.	Keep medicines locked up in childproof bottles.
Burns	Child falls on electric fire.	Put burned area into cold water, take child to hospital.	Have a fixed guard over fires.
Drowning	Child slips under water.	Mouth-to-mouth resuscitation, take child to hospital.	Supervise child all the time.

Prevention of accidents involving the elderly

Sometimes old people cannot see as well as they used to and they are more likely to fall over. Their bones are very brittle and a fall usually results in a broken bone. Any cuts on their skin usually take much longer to heal and can become infected. Elderly people suffer from the cold which slows down how quickly they react to danger, so they are more likely to have an accident.

Here is a list of some of the things which you could do to help prevent elderly people having an accident:

- put guards on all fires
- keep clothes away from heaters
- get the wiring of all electrical appliances checked
- warm the bed with an electric blanket or hot water bottle
- encourage the person to wear layers of clothes in cold weather
- make sure the person has regular meals each day, especially a hot breakfast
- make sure someone calls in every day to visit and check the person is alright, especially in winter
- find out if extra help is available from Social Security to help with heating bills.

A new scheme to help the elderly

Some local authorities have set up a scheme so that elderly people can get help in an emergency. The person wears a pendant chain around their neck. The pendant has an electronic device which if pressed, will automatically make the telephone dial a number in an 'emergency centre' and help can be sent immediately. This device is especially useful when a person may have broken a bone and be unable to move.

---

1 What should you do if a small child is choking after swallowing a small object?
2 Why should you keep plastic bags away from children?
3 How can you prevent children falling down stairs?
4 What is the effect of cold weather on elderly people?
5 List three things you should do to prevent an elderly person from having an accident.
6 Why is it important that someone visits an old person every day especially in winter?
7 Investigate the possibilities of visiting an elderly person near where you live.

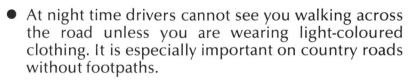

Unit 14 Road Safety

Whenever you use the roads, either as a pedestrian, cyclist or driver, there are certain rules you should remember for your own safety and the safety of other road users. All the information you should know is contained in a useful booklet called the **Highway Code**. This booklet, available from bookshops, contains all the basic hints, points of law, road signs and signals for cyclists, pedestrians, drivers, motorcyclists, and people with animals on the road. You must learn the main points in the Highway Code when you begin to ride a motorbike or drive a car.

Some of the main points which relate to pedestrians, cyclists and drivers from the Highway Code, are described below.

Dangers to pedestrians

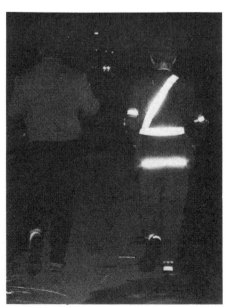

- At night time drivers cannot see you walking across the road unless you are wearing light-coloured clothing. It is especially important on country roads without footpaths.

  Remember: at night, wear something light.

- Make sure you always walk on the pavement or footpath. If you are walking along a road without a path you should face the traffic approaching you.
- When you are walking along a road with a child, make sure that you walk between the child and the traffic.
- When you want to cross the road use a proper pedestrian crossing, traffic lights, subways, footbridges or central islands.
- A driver is not able to see you in time to stop if you cross the road from in between parked cars.

Zebra crossings

You have priority on a zebra crossing only when a car has stopped for you. Cars need a lot of time and space to stop in. They will not be able to stop if you step out in front of them.

Pelican crossings or signal-controlled crossings

Wait for the 'Green Man' to appear before you start to cross. If the Green Man is 'flashing' you do not have time to start crossing the road.

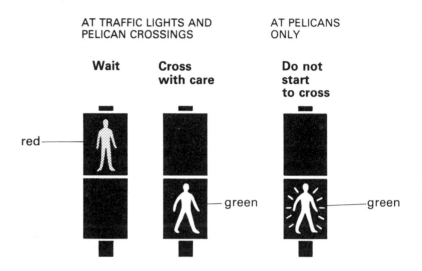

Green Cross Code

You are responsible for your own safety. You need to learn and use the Green Cross Code.

- Before you cross the road stop at the kerb, look right, look left and look right again
- Walk straight across the road, not at an angle
- Do not run across the road as you may fall over
- Remember 3 out of 4 pedestrians killed or seriously injured are under 15 or over 60. Don't let it be you.

Dangers to cyclists

- Make sure your bike is in good condition. Check brakes, tyres, lamps and rear reflector. Many cyclists are killed or injured because other road users cannot see them.

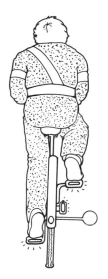

Make sure you can be seen.

- Always look behind you before pulling out, or turning right or left.
- Only ride in single file on busy or narrow roads.
- Hold the handlebar and keep your feet on the pedals at all times.
- Make sure your bike is balanced and don't carry passengers unless you have a specially adapted bike.

Wear bright reflective clothing especially at night. It is possible to buy armbands or chest bands to wear which are reflective. Reflective discs attached to bicycle wheels are also very useful.

Dangers to drivers and passengers

- You must keep your car in good condition. Check tyres, brakes, lights, steering and visibility.
- Always wear a safety belt and make sure any children are safely strapped in.

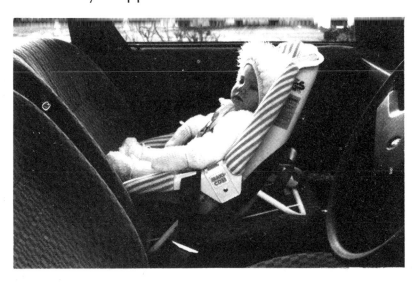

The safest way of carrying a baby in a car.

'Drinking and driving'

When you are responsible for driving a car you should not drink alcohol. Drinking alcohol slows down your judgement and reaction time. This means that you will react more slowly in an emergency. You could easily hit a person and kill or injure them. You could also hit an object such as a lamppost and seriously injure or kill yourself. One in three of the drivers who are killed in road accidents have been drinking alcohol just prior to their accident.

The legal limit for drinking and driving is three units of alcohol, which is about three standard drinks, that is 1½ pints of beer, 3 glasses of wine, or 3 glasses of spirit such as whisky or gin.

The legal limit for driving is three units of alcohol. It doesn't take many drinks to reach this limit.

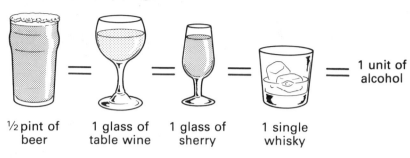

½ pint of beer = 1 glass of table wine = 1 glass of sherry = 1 single whisky = 1 unit of alcohol

It takes over an hour for your body to 'lose' one standard drink, but this depends on whether you are male or female and on your weight. If you have drunk too much alcohol you will need to give your body time to break down the alcohol so that the effects wear off. If you drink at lunchtime you may still be affected in the evening. It is much better to walk or get a taxi, than to drive when you have drunk too much alcohol and risk injuring yourself or someone else. People who depend on their driving licence for their work find that life becomes very difficult and expensive if they lose their licence through a conviction for driving while over the legal limit.

The best safety precaution is not to drink any alcohol if you are driving. It is now socially acceptable to refuse alcoholic drinks when you are driving. Most people respect someone who says 'No alcohol, I'm driving'.

1 Why should you wear bright coloured clothing at night?
2 When should you start to cross when using a pelican crossing?
3 What is the 'Green Cross Code'?
4 What should you check before using your bike?
5 Why should you not drink alcohol when you are driving?
6 How much beer makes you 'over the limit'?
7 What should you do if you have drunk too much and have to get home?
8 Why is the Highway Code a useful booklet to read?

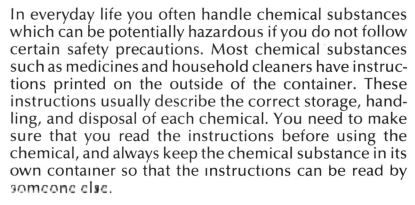

Unit 15 Safety with Chemicals

In everyday life you often handle chemical substances which can be potentially hazardous if you do not follow certain safety precautions. Most chemical substances such as medicines and household cleaners have instructions printed on the outside of the container. These instructions usually describe the correct storage, handling, and disposal of each chemical. You need to make sure that you read the instructions before using the chemical, and always keep the chemical substance in its own container so that the instructions can be read by someone else.

The chart on the next page summarizes the main points of safety which you should know about storage, handling and disposal of drugs, compressed gases, insecticides, aerosols, bleaches and disinfectants.

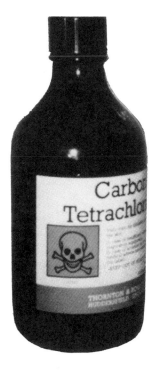

1 Where should all drugs be kept?
2 What precautions should always be taken when changing a gas cartridge?
3 What two precautions should you take when handling insecticides?
4 What should you never do to an empty aerosol can?
5 What should you do if you get bleach or disinfectant on your skin, or even worse, if you should swallow some?

Substance	Storage	Handling	Disposal
Drugs	Keep all medicines out of reach of young children. Where possible keep all medicines in a locked cupboard.	Make sure you read the label on the bottle. Do not take more than the recommended amount.	Use the medicines before the expiry date. Flush away unused medicines or tablets.
Compressed gases	Store below 50°C in a dry place. Keep out of reach of children.	Never use near a naked flame. Only change a gas cartridge when it is empty and only outside.	Do not pierce the can or put it on a fire.
Insecticides	Keep in a dry cool place. Keep in labelled containers only. Keep out of reach of children or animals.	Follow the instructions. Wear protective clothing especially boots and gloves. Wash your hands after using. Keep pets away from treated areas.	Dispose carefully of any unused chemicals in sealed plastic bags.
Aerosols	Keep away from young children. Protect from sunlight and keep at below 50°C.	Follow the instructions. Do not spray near a flame or at people's faces.	Do not pierce the can or put it on a fire.
Bleaches and disinfectants	Store upright in a cool place, away from children. Do not remove the label and do not put the chemical into another bottle.	Do not mix with other cleaning fluids. Wash off skin or eyes with plenty of water. If swallowed, drink plenty of water.	Pour away down a drain with plenty of cold water.

Index

organs 7, 18, 48
ovaries 26, 86
oviduct (egg tube) 26, 28, 74
ovulation 26–7
oxygen 8, 12–4, 15–7, 28, 30, 84

pancreas 10–1
parasites 76–81
paraffin (oil) heaters 91, 97
pasteurization 61, 80
pedestrians 109–10
pelican crossings 110
penicillin 74
penis 27–8, 39, 73–4, 75
periods 26–7
Pest Control Officer 67
physical handicaps 53–5
placenta 28
plaque 35
plasma 15
platelets 15
plugs, wiring of 102–3
polio 54, 70
pollution
    air 84–6
    noise 82–4
    radiation 86–7
posture 21
pregnancy 27, 28, 49, 50, 54, 86, 98
preservatives 60
proteins 8, 10, 25, 30–1
Public Health Authority 80
pupil 24

quarantine 80

radiation 60, 82, 86–7
rashes 48, 68–9, 73, 74
rats 58, 65, 66–7, 76
reasoning 21–2
rectum 11, 74, 78
Red Cross, British 99, 105
reflex actions 21, 22–3
refrigeration 58–9
relaxation 34, 42, 44–6
reproductive system 8, 9, 26–9, 68, 72–4
respiration (breathing) 12–4, 21, 105

respiratory system 8, 9, 12–4
resuscitation 105, 107
retina 24
ribs 13, 14, 19
road safety 109–10
roughage (fibre) 12, 30–1
rubella (German measles) 28, 54, 70

STD clinics 72, 75
saliva 8, 65, 75
salivary glands 8
Salmonella 62, 63
salt 25
salting 60
Samaritans 42
scabies 78
scalds 99
'sell-by' date 62
semen 27–8, 75
sense cells 21–5
sensory nerves 21–5
serum 71
sex organs 26–7, 39, 73–5, 79
sexual intercourse 28, 72, 75
sexually transmitted diseases (STD) 72–6
silica 85–6
silicosis 85
skeletal system 8, 9, 18–21
skin rash 48, 68–9, 73, 74
skull 18, 19
sleep 33–4
sleeping sickness 76
small intestine 10–1
smallpox 71
smoking 17, 28, 49, 85, 86, 92
smoking of food 60
sodium 31
solvents 52
soot 84
sperm 27–8, 86
sperm duct 27, 74
spinal cord 21–3
St John's Ambulance Brigade 99, 105
starch 10, 30–1
sterility 74, 86
stimulus 22, 43
stomach 10–1
stomach ulcers 43, 50

Acknowledgements

The author and publishers are grateful to the following for permission to reproduce copyright photographs:
pp. 14, 19 (both), 74, 78 (right), Department of Medical Illustration, St. Bartholomew's Hospital; p. 15, Biophoto Associates; pp. 23, 30, 34, 36, 37, 48, 52 (top left), 57, 58 (top left), 67, 81, 85, 91, 96, 113, Barnabys Picture Library; p. 35, Argentum/Science Photo Library; p. 56, Will McIntyre/ Science Photo Library; p. 77 (both), Cath Wadforth/ Science Photo Library; p. 78 (bottom left), Sinclair Stammers/Science Photo Library; p. 52 (bottom left), Will Green; p. 58, J Sainsbury PLC; p. 61, National Dairy Council; pp. 65, 66, S. Dalton/NHPA; p. 79, A. Bannister/ NHPA; p. 80, Meat and Livestock Commission; p. 87, United Kingdom Atomic Energy Authority; p. 89, British Cleaning Council; pp. 109, 111, Royal Society for the Prevention of Accidents (RoSPA)

and to the following for permission to reproduce copyright material:
p. 75 (AIDS leaflet cover), HMSO; p. 93 (fire prevention leaflet), Central Office of Information (COI).

Cover photograph by Chris Gilbert

Technical artwork by RDL Artset

Biological drawings by Nancy Sutcliffe

Cartoons by John Erasmus